Living with Baria

Living with Bariatric Surgery: Managing Your Mind and Your Weight aims to help those who are considering bariatric surgery develop a psychological understanding of their eating behaviour and the changes needed in order to make surgery successful. It is also a resource for those who have undergone surgery to help them adapt to the physical, psychological and relationship adjustments that occur.

Whilst the benefits of bariatric surgery are significant, the psychological challenges it presents for patients have been overlooked. This book will help patients develop a realistic view of bariatric surgery and the changes required. It incorporates the real-life experiences of people who have had bariatric surgery, showing how they have responded to the psychological and behavioural changes after surgery, and also features helpful psychoeducation, exercises and strategies to facilitate reflection and learning.

Living with Bariatric Surgery will be an essential guide for anyone considering, preparing for or recovering from bariatric surgery, as well as health professionals working with these clients.

Denise Ratcliffe is a Consultant Clinical Psychologist who has worked in bariatric surgery for the past 10 years. She is the psychology lead for bariatric surgery at Chelsea and Westminster Hospital and Phoenix Health, UK. She is also Head of Clinical Health Psychology at Chelsea and Westminster Hospital.

Living with Bariatric Surgery

Managing Your Mind and Your Weight

Denise Ratcliffe

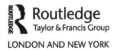
Routledge
Taylor & Francis Group

LONDON AND NEW YORK

First published 2018
by Routledge
2 Park Square, Milton Park, Abingdon, Oxon OX14 4RN

and by Routledge
711 Third Avenue, New York, NY 10017

Routledge is an imprint of the Taylor & Francis Group, an informa business

British Library Cataloguing in Publication Data
A catalogue record for this book is available from the British Library

Library of Congress Cataloging in Publication Data
A catalog record for this book has been requested

ISBN: 978-1-138-21711-9 (hbk)
ISBN: 978-1-138-21712-6 (pbk)
ISBN: 978-1-315-39830-3 (ebk)

Typeset in Times New Roman
by Swales & Willis Ltd, Exeter, Devon, UK

Contents

Acknowledgements

I would like to thank the patients who have generously shared their lives and experiences and enabled me to develop an understanding of the psychological aspects of bariatric surgery. I hope that I have achieved my aim of capturing their experiences and learning in order to help others going through this process.

I would also like to acknowledge the incredible and inspirational bariatric surgery teams at Chelsea and Westminster Hospital and Phoenix Health. I would particularly like to thank Kelli Edmiston, Nuala Davison, Kathy McCabe and Hayley Pluckwell.

On a personal note, I would like to dedicate this book to Derek Staton, my husband and soulmate. You are my home.

I would also like to thank my parents and sister for their support and encouragement, and for simply being the most decent, kind human beings.

Introduction

Bariatric surgery is the most effective way to lose weight for individuals who are very overweight. It can provide an exit route from a lifelong struggle of trying to lose weight and going through endless cycles of yo-yo dieting. It has the potential to be life-changing and life-saving. However, it is important to be realistic about the benefits of bariatric surgery and the likely challenges and skills required to achieve long-term success. The surgical operations themselves take less than a couple of hours, but the changes and commitment to make the surgery work last a lifetime. The surgery is just a tool. There is an increasing awareness of the role that psychological and behavioural factors play in influencing what happens to people after surgery and whether they achieve their goals:

> A welcome and overdue advance in bariatric surgical practice over the past 10 years has been the recognition that if we are to empower patients to get the best from their surgery, we have to adopt a holistic approach that acknowledges that surgery alone cannot guarantee good outcomes.
>
> Professor David Kerrigan,
> Consultant Bariatric Surgeon, Phoenix Health

It is important to update your mind and your behaviour at the same time that your stomach changes! This book is about helping you to make sure your new stomach and mind are working together, and that they are both working towards the same goal of weight loss. You are planning a surgical intervention on your stomach. This book provides the intervention for your brain.

Bariatric surgery is a life-changing but complex psychological process to undergo. The benefits of surgery and weight loss are numerous, but it does create a different set of issues to negotiate and manage. This book aims to help you make the changes and adjustments required to achieve a successful outcome following surgery in terms of weight loss and your wider life. It will help you prepare for surgery and aims to equip you with the skills to avoid and manage the pitfalls and obstacles you may face. The book is based on my clinical practice of working in the area for 10 years and coming into contact with hundreds of patients who have been through the process of having bariatric surgery. It also draws on the experiences of people who have had surgery and includes feedback from them about the changes they have experienced and what they have found helpful in managing these.

How effective is bariatric surgery?

Bariatric surgery is the most effective treatment for obesity that currently exists. It has the potential to be life-saving and life-changing. The best-known study of bariatric surgery compared the weight loss of those who had bariatric surgery with those that tried to manage their weight using typical diets over a 20-year period. The results of this study are compelling as they show that the weight of those who dieted over this period of time only changed by an average of 3% (either up or down), showing that their weight loss did not significantly change. However, those who had bariatric surgery, particularly gastric bypass, lost an average of 25–32% of their weight over this time period (Sjostrom 2013).

To put this into context, a man who weighed 150kg would have lost 45kg (30%) in the 20-year period after surgery, whereas if he did not have surgery then his weight would have changed (this could be either up or down) by an average of 4.5kg during this 20-year period. This compelling evidence clearly demonstrates that bariatric surgery can lead to many physical and psychological improvements.

These include:

Physical

    Diabetes

    Sleep apnoea

    Hypertension

    Polycystic ovarian syndrome

Fertility

Joint pain

Improved energy

Reduced breathlessness.

Psychological

Reduced depression and anxiety

Improved quality of life

Improved self-esteem and confidence

Improved body image

Reduction in binge eating (short term at least).

How much weight do people lose after bariatric surgery?

Most people lose most of their weight in the first two years after surgery, with most weight loss occurring in the first 12 months. This one- to two-year period following surgery presents a window of opportunity to have a different experience of weight loss and to make changes that lead to sustainable weight loss. Research shows that people vary significantly in terms of how much weight they lose, with some people starting to regain weight at around 6–12 months after surgery.

The way that weight loss is usually defined after bariatric surgery is through calculating the percentage of excess weight loss (referred to as %EWL) – this refers to the percentage of weight lost between your weight before surgery and what you would weigh if you had a body mass index (BMI) of 25. It is important to understand this as the research provides information about the average %EWL following different bariatric operations. Your bariatric service will be able to calculate what they would expect your weight to be after surgery if you make the required changes and stick to the post-op plan.

The average %EWL following different procedures are shown below:

Roux en y gastric bypass   75%

Sleeve gastrectomy   65%

Gastric band   50%

	Expected weight following bypass	Expected weight following sleeve gastrectomy	Expected weight following gastric band
Man, Height 5'11 Pre op weight 150kg BMI 46.3	98kg	102kg	116kg
Female Height 5'6 Pre op weight 120kg BMI 43	82kg	87kg	95kg

Figure 0.1 Examples of average predicted changes in weight following bariatric surgery

This means that even after bariatric surgery, your BMI is still likely to be in the overweight range and at least 25% over BMI 25. This is considered a successful outcome after bariatric surgery, although it sometimes differs from what individuals hope or expect to lose.

Whilst it is clear that bariatric surgery is the most effective way of losing and maintaining weight loss for those who have severe weight problems, it is important to be aware that evidence shows there is the potential for weight regain – approximately 20% of people will regain a significant amount of weight after surgery. The difference in weight loss between people is influenced by the extent to which they manage their emotional health and their ability to stick to the eating plan. This is why it is so important to be realistic about the fact that surgery is just one of the tools required, and that you will need to implement, and maintain, significant behaviour changes in order to maintain weight loss and avoid regaining weight.

Weight regain is often devastating for people and often leads to poor mental health – it can lead to feelings of shame and failure, and this can sometimes trigger problem eating again. On the other hand, poor emotional and mental health are often the cause of weight regain, too. This is why people often see a psychologist before and after bariatric surgery to help them prepare beforehand and to cope with the changes and adjustments following surgery.

Bariatric surgery is often a landmark moment in people's lives, one where the potential benefits are life-changing but the consequences of it not having the desired outcome can be devastating.

Why is psychology an important part of bariatric surgery?

Surgeons who have worked in bariatric surgery for many years increasingly recognise the importance of behavioural and psychological factors:

The bariatric operations do not, and cannot, work in isolation of patient motivation and their underlying psychology. The role of psychological factors in bariatric patients remains critically important. Patients will not have successful weight outcomes if they are not behaviourally prepared to incorporate changes that can minimise weight regain. Many patients will already have a complex psychological background in terms of their relationship with food, eating patterns and body image. These all need effectively addressing before surgery is even contemplated, as psychological factors regularly impact on weight loss and coping after surgery. The bariatric surgical procedure serves as a tool to induce weight loss; however, for true bariatric success, psychological factors at all stages of the patient journey require continued thought and action to achieve a successful outcome.

Mr Evangelos Efthimiou,
Consultant Bariatric Surgeon, Chelsea
and Westminster Hospital, UK

Bariatric surgery is obviously different to other types of surgery where you have an operation which fixes or cures the problem. With bariatric surgery, the operation is just a small part of the process – the psychological and behavioural changes that run alongside the operation are necessary to make it work.

I now realise the psychological bit is 75% – most of us have an unhealthy relationship with food. That's not a physical thing, it's psychological, and the operation doesn't change that. The physical operation is a tool and it does work, but it won't work unless you get your head working with it. That's why people put weight on again because they haven't changed their relationship with food.

GM – initially had a gastric band with minimal
weight loss and then had a bypass

Aside from the behaviour changes required to make bariatric surgery effective, there are other psychological adjustments that occur as a result of rapid weight loss – a changing relationship with food, body image and relationship changes.

The surgery is just a milestone but all of the difficulties I've had have come from my head – struggling with how you look and how you feel. I don't know how anyone could go through such a dramatic transformation and not have some challenges along the way when you try to get your head around it. Friends sometimes aren't able to help because they have no idea about the process and they are just like bystanders. Just knowing that there will be struggles and there will be some that you know are coming and that you can deal with and then there will be some that are frightening and overwhelming that you didn't expect. I can't see how anyone can go through this kind of process . . . it's a process of disengaging from your relationship with food . . . its really challenging. The way I think and feel about food is so completely different and it will never be like it used to be again. I think of this post-op phase as a foundation for the rest of my life.

AM, 6 months post bypass

There are three main areas where psychological factors play an important role in bariatric surgery. These are:

- pre-existing psychological difficulties that people have experienced that may influence how they may cope
- psychological difficulties that people have experienced that affect their eating and relationship with food
- psychological difficulties that arise as a result of the bariatric surgery (and all its consequences) itself.

Most people will experience an issue in at least one of these areas, and this can affect how much weight they lose after bariatric surgery and how they cope. Remember it's not just about weight loss: it's about how you feel emotionally, too.

As we go through each of these areas in a bit more detail, consider whether there are particular areas you identify with.

Pre-existing psychological difficulties that may affect eating/weight problems or coping

These are the psychological difficulties and experiences that people bring with them to the bariatric process which can influence how they respond and cope. For example, psychological difficulties such as depression which can affect motivation, planning and confidence levels.

There are higher rates of psychological difficulties amongst people who have obesity. This includes mood problems such as depression and anxiety as well as low self-esteem and binge eating disorder. There are also much higher rates of adverse childhood experiences including abuse and neglect. There is a wide spectrum of psychological difficulties that vary in severity, intensity and the impact they may have on a person and how they cope with surgery.

We know that many factors contribute to obesity including genetic and hormonal factors, psychological issues, socio-economic and environmental factors. The psychological component (e.g. emotional eating, depression) that causes obesity will vary between each individual – for some people, it is only a small part, whereas for others, it is a major contributor. If you imagine a pie chart of factors that have caused an individual's weight problems, the slice that relates to psychological factors is going to be much larger for some people than others.

It is important to be clear that I am not suggesting that everyone who has weight issues has mental health or psychological problems. Many people are under the impression that people who are obese have undiagnosed psychological problems and that these are the cause of their obesity. Whilst the research tells us that those people who have mental health problems are more likely to have problems with obesity than the general population, in reality, it's a two-way street between psychological problems and obesity. The extent to which psychological factors contribute towards an individual's weight varies significantly between people; however, the experience of struggling with weight and dieting clearly has a psychological toll.

Just because someone has mental health problems doesn't necessarily mean that bariatric surgery isn't an option that should be considered. In fact, for many people, surgery can actually lead to many psychological improvements. It can be a psychological intervention as well as a surgical intervention. However, the evidence tells us that those people who have mental health difficulties are at higher risk of losing less weight than those without mental health difficulties (Kinzl et al., 2006). Whilst this research indicates that having mental health problems may put someone at risk of having a less good outcome after surgery, it doesn't necessarily mean that they shouldn't have surgery: it's about being aware of the risk and thinking about how this can be managed so it has less impact. It is important to have a discussion with the psychologist and bariatric team about the impact any mental health issues may have on your eating, how you manage daily activities and how you might cope with change. It is also about putting a plan in place so that if your mental health changes then you know what to do and who to call upon to manage it quickly and effectively.

Eating patterns and behaviours that are rooted in psychological issues

We know that many people use food as a way of managing their emotions or coping with difficult situations or feelings. This means that we start to believe that food is an emotional cure or tonic, and we base our behaviour on this. Eating problems can be associated with certain psychological problems, too – for example, if someone is depressed, they may overeat to lift their mood or may eat more convenience take-away foods as their motivation is affected by depression.

There can be all sorts of reasons why these patterns develop – sometimes people learn early in life that food is a comfort if they are feeling upset or stressed. The underlying difficulties causing emotional problems remain, but the way of coping with them creates another problem.

We know that there are much higher rates of difficult traumatic experiences and abuse in people with weight issues compared to the general population. We collected information from over 1,400 people seeking bariatric surgery in our service, and 25% of them said that they had experienced trauma which they felt had affected their eating behaviour. Food can be a source of comfort and soothing, or distraction from problems.

If you have used food as a way of coping with difficult emotions or situations, then it can be challenging and unsettling to not have that available as an option after surgery.

> It is really important to understand your relationship with food before and what it might mean to take that away. You have to be prepared to put a safety net in place for when you can no longer rely on food anymore.
>
> ER, 18 months post bypass

It is far better to take some time to develop your understanding of why this eating behaviour happens and develop some skills to find other ways of managing emotions, before surgery.

Psychological and behavioural issues that arise from bariatric surgery

The rapid and dramatic weight loss that often happens after bariatric surgery can create a different set of psychological adjustments and challenges, for example, changes in your relationship with food, body image, your relationships and so on. Most people will experience these adjustments and changes after surgery – whilst they are often positive, they are challenging because they are unfamiliar. There can also be more complex difficulties that people experience. Some examples include regretting the surgery (especially if they have complications after surgery and can't progress with their eating) or experiencing major problems with excess skin. Other issues may include disappointment with weight loss and unmet expectations about the impact of weight loss on their wider life.

In this book, we will cover each of these areas and provide the information and the tools to help you get through the process. Part I of the book focuses on preparation for surgery, and Part II focuses on life after surgery.

The first half of the book focuses on increasing your knowledge about the changes required for bariatric surgery to work, helping to build your awareness and recognising eating patterns and traps that need to be overcome.

The second half of the book focuses on adjustments that are experienced following surgery in relation to weight, eating, emotional health, body image and relationships. The book will outline some of the typical changes and adjustments that need to be navigated as well as highlighting pitfalls to avoid.

References

Kinzl, J.F., et al. 2006. Psychosocial predictors of weight loss after bariatric surgery. *Obesity Surgery*, *16* (12), 1609–14. doi:10.1381/096089206779319301

Sjostrom, L. 2013. Review of the key results from the Swedish Obese Subjects (SOS) trial prospective controlled intervention study of bariatric surgery. *Journal of Internal Medicine*, 273 (3), 219–234. doi:10.1111/joim.12012

Part I

Getting ready for bariatric surgery

The first part of the book focuses on making changes in preparation for bariatric surgery. This involves developing new habits, addressing emotional eating patterns and creating foundations for a smooth transition into life after surgery.

Chapter 1

Developing a balanced and realistic view of bariatric surgery

Most people who are considering bariatric surgery feel that they have exhausted all other options to lose weight and that bariatric surgery is their only, and last, option remaining. They have usually struggled with their weight for many years and have tried many diets over these years. Most people are able to lose weight when they are on a diet but find it impossible to maintain this weight loss. This often leads to a pattern of yo-yo dieting of weight loss and weight regain (usually with extra weight), and this is mentally and physically stressful. Bariatric surgery presents an opportunity to make positive changes and improve your health as demonstrated in the quotation below:

> Bariatric surgery has led to a fundamental change for the better. From feeling incredibly dark, unengaged and uninspired with no energy and lack of purpose to the exact opposite . . . I now have too much energy and I'm much more confident and comfortable in myself. I'm now more able to engage and do things that I never thought possible before.
>
> TG, 16 months post bypass

Whilst the positive aspects of bariatric surgery are clear, it does also create a different set of challenges to navigate and negotiate your way through. It is important to have some awareness of these, as they are not necessarily issues that one might predict.

We did a survey of people who had bariatric surgery in our clinic and we asked the following questions:

1   What have been the positive aspects of having bariatric surgery for you?
2   What are the challenges or difficulties that you have experienced after bariatric surgery?
3   Would you recommend bariatric surgery to a friend in a similar situation?

The main improvements that people reported were improved confidence, improved health and being able to do things that were previously unmanageable. The main challenges described were body image, excess skin, difficulties adjusting to eating and relationship issues. A total of 95% said that they would recommend bariatric surgery to a friend in a similar situation, and 5% said that they would "maybe" recommend surgery. Interestingly, nobody who completed the survey said that they would not recommend surgery to a friend in a similar situation (Ratcliffe et al. 2012).

Each person will have their own individual path leading up to, through and beyond bariatric surgery. Although the surgical operations are the same, the issues that you have to deal with before and those which arise afterwards will be unique to you and depend on your previous experiences, your problem-solving and coping skills and support. This will inevitably affect how you cope and what you get from the surgery.

It is important to think about and work on the psychological aspect of bariatric surgery because:

*   the operation itself is only a tool, and you need to implement and maintain long-term eating changes to avoid poor weight loss.
*   the adjustments following surgery can be challenging in terms of managing changes in your eating and weight, body image changes, staying on track and avoiding weight regain, etc.

Bariatric surgery is part of the answer, not the complete solution

Bariatric surgery is only a tool – it is just a more effective one than dieting alone for people who are very overweight. In fact, the surgery itself is only one of the tools you need in your toolkit in order to manage your weight. This becomes increasingly important over time. The surgery provides a window of opportunity to make changes that will then become lifelong.

For me, the psychological bit of surgery has been fundamental. The surgery has allowed me to have a break along with a period of rapid weight loss . . . that's the initial bit that comes for free with the surgery. You are always going to have that dramatic weight loss for a few months and so that gives you the break to allow you to address your relationship with food. You've got everything you need to climb up the ladder. You've got that break from the immediate urges and the needs to eat certain foods that the surgery gives you . . . that's quite a short period of about 10 weeks before you are back to normal foods. I didn't feel hungry during that time. The psychological distance that you get is crucial. Your body and your mind come together to be able to regulate what you are eating. The psychological aspect is more to do with the patterns of behaviour you had before and after surgery; you feel you've got the strength and the distance to address them.

TG, 16 months post bypass

It is the individual's behaviour that activates and puts the power into the surgery. If you imagine someone cycling on a bicycle, they will continue to travel without needing to pedal whilst they are going downhill, but over time, they will run out of steam and they will need to pedal to stay upright and to keep moving. This is the same with surgery – initially you are likely to get some "automatic" weight loss for the first few months after surgery, but this slows over time and the person's behaviour becomes crucially important in determining what happens next with their weight. The changes you make alongside the operation are crucial: it's a partnership – one without the other reduces the power of the intervention and its effectiveness.

The operation is a helping hand, it's not the complete answer. For some people, it might get their weight down but they will still have to do things to maintain that weight loss and stop it creeping up. I think people need to know it's an additional tool, it's a headstart but you've still got to change your mindset. I lost weight afterwards but I've put some back on because I didn't make all the changes I needed to – I've really had to accept that I've got to work with it.

NR, regained some weight after bypass

In the following chapters, you will find out more about the eating and activity behaviours that need to happen alongside the surgery for long-term weight loss. Most people have had the experience of putting a lot of effort into diets and weight loss before surgery, but the results tend to be minimal or short-lived. There is an imbalance between the amount of effort and the results. However, after bariatric surgery there seems to be a more reliable and fairer relationship between the effort put into making changes following surgery and the subsequent weight loss. This creates a virtuous cycle whereby positive changes lead to positive results which then motivate people to continue because they feel it's working and it's worthwhile.

What do you have to do to make surgery successful?

It is important to step back and honestly ask yourself whether you are prepared to make the compromises needed after bariatric surgery. It is easy for people to quickly reassure themselves by saying, "It will be fine", but it is really important to stop and think it through – if you have surgery, what will you miss or not be able to do in future, and is that going to be manageable for you? Is it worth it? Are the losses and changes going to be outweighed by the benefits for you?

It is important to be aware that if you smoke or drink alcohol regularly, you will be expected to stop for a significant period of time before surgery.

Those people who are successful after bariatric surgery generally do the following:

- Eat regularly
- Eat small portions
- Plan meals
- Prioritise eating certain food types, e.g. protein
- Follow the same eating routine
- Are highly aware of their eating
- Avoid eating certain foods
- Avoid unhelpful eating patterns such as grazing and binge eating
- Avoid alcohol
- Don't smoke
- Follow the "golden rules" – specific bariatric eating techniques (e.g. eating and drinking separately)
- Take multivitamin and supplements regularly
- Exercise regularly
- Attend regular follow-up appointments.

Anybody looking at this list of behaviours may feel overwhelmed and daunted! Some of these behaviours and changes you may already be doing and any others you can tackle over time. If you focus and work hard at these fundamental behaviours, they will become your new habits. This means they will become less effortful over time. This book aims to help you start to develop strategies and put behaviours in place that will make these changes much easier.

It is important to be aware of what bariatric surgery will and won't do for you so that you make a rational and informed choice about whether it is the right option for you at this point in your life.

Review of common myths

Weight loss after bariatric surgery is guaranteed

It is highly unusual for people not to lose weight after surgery, but it is possible to lose less weight than expected or regain weight. The differences in weight loss start to emerge at just six months (Courcoulas et al. 2013). This is around the time that the honeymoon period ends and your role in making surgery work really kicks in.

Bariatric surgery will stop me from eating

You will still have to make the choices and decisions about what to eat, when to eat and how to eat. You are likely to get more feedback from your stomach after your operation – for example, stronger signals of fullness and pain or other symptoms if you eat foods that are not suitable. Some people find these signals helpful as it can help them work out what to avoid. However, despite these signals, it is still you who decides what to put into your stomach. Don't forget – the brain is stronger than the stomach!

I won't put any weight on again after having bariatric surgery

Approximately 20–25% of people will have either insufficient weight loss or will put on a significant amount of weight after bariatric surgery (Sheets et al. 2014). Sadly, the operation is not a guarantee of permanent weight loss. That is the reason why adherence to the post-op bariatric eating and activity plan is so important, because this is what helps you to maintain weight loss.

I will repeat the yo-yo pattern and put all the weight back on again

The evidence is that people generally lose more weight and keep more of it off in the longer term compared to any other method of weight loss. There is some research which shows there is a natural trend towards slight weight regain two years after surgery (Courcoulas et al. 2013). This is very different to the previous pattern of regaining all the lost weight plus more. As discussed earlier, some patients regain weight or don't lose as much as expected, but it's rare (although possible) for people to put all their weight back on again.

I will never be able to enjoy food again

The aim is for you to be able to enjoy eating food after surgery, just in smaller portions – it is about developing a healthy relationship with food. This involves moving away from the dieting mindset which tends to lead to "all-or-nothing" thinking about food. This leads people to ricochet from feeling deprived to losing control of their eating. After bariatric surgery, we want to move away from the extremes of feeling deprived of food and overeating (this is typical of the dieting mindset) and we want to find a middle ground. This involves discovering ways of consciously having small and limited amounts of food that you enjoy and getting the maximum pleasure out of that experience.

Bariatric surgery is a quick fix/cheat

Absolutely not. You will still need to actively manage your eating and activity behaviours – as you can see from the list of behaviours outlined, there is a lot to focus on and implement, and these don't happen automatically or overnight. This is why it is important to prepare for surgery and view it as a process of change rather than a single intervention.

Dieting can affect your self-confidence

Past experiences of dieting can impact someone's confidence about their ability to make changes or to succeed at weight loss. Bariatric surgery can seem like a daunting, unimaginable process or alternatively, sometimes people dismiss the relevance of the behaviour change aspects believing that the surgery will do all the work.

Most people who are considering bariatric surgery have struggled with their weight for years and years and have usually tried most diets available. The pattern of yo-yo dieting, with weight loss followed by weight regain plus extra weight, is usually a familiar and painful experience. Some people feel ashamed about "failing" to lose weight and describe "needing" to have bariatric surgery as a sign that they have "given up the battle" and that they do not have the internal resources or strength to manage their weight and therefore need an external "fix".

There can be a sense of embarrassment and shame about having surgery to help with something that we are led to believe we "should" be able to manage ourselves if only we were motivated or strong-willed enough. However, we need to turn this idea on its head – obesity is classed as a disease: it is not a lifestyle choice. If you step back and think about it, how would you respond to a friend who told you that they were trying to access the most evidence-based treatment for their physical health condition? Would you criticise or support them?

The fact that people have often persisted for so long at trying to lose weight is remarkable. If this were any other area, we would be praising someone for their dedication and determination despite the odds of achieving their goal being stacked against them. Weight loss is often presented as easy and quick if only someone has the willpower and motivation, yet this does not capture the true picture. A study by Fildes et al. (2015) looked at people's weight over a nine-year period and found that if someone had a BMI over 40 (which puts them in the severely obese range), then men had a 1 in 1290 chance and women had a 1 in 677 chance of getting into the healthy weight range (BMI between 20–25). Furthermore, they showed that about 60% of people put weight on again after losing weight. This demonstrates the reality of the challenge that people face with losing and maintaining weight loss.

We know that some people have a strong genetic predisposition to put weight on, and therefore, some people have a bigger challenge in managing their weight compared to others. In fact, obesity is now classified as a disease by the World Health Organisation. The mismatch between the impression we are given about how easy and simple it is to lose weight versus the reality that most people experience often leads to a sense of failure, shame and frustration. These views can contribute to people feeling that they have failed and affect their confidence when thinking about making changes in future.

What makes bariatric surgery different to previous diets?

First, the eating plan before and after bariatric surgery is not about being on a diet. Diets usually involve following a set of imposed rules, cutting out certain foods and feeling hungry; the combination of these usually tends to lead to the opposite effect as cravings build. There's nothing like telling yourself that you can't have ice-cream to make you desperately want it! Also, people tend to alternate between going "on" a diet and then "off" a diet, whereas bariatric surgery is about establishing a long-term eating plan that works with your new stomach.

The quotations below, from people who have had bariatric surgery, explain the differences they have noticed between eating after bariatric surgery and their previous diets.

I think I've probably tried every diet known to man. I've always lost weight but I've only ever ended up heavier at the end. I think when I had surgery I was so desperate to be in a different place . . . I was 26 stone [165.1kg] and could hardly move . . . I felt completely lost. I lost massive amounts after surgery . . . about 10 stone [63.5kg] and my life was absolutely transformed. It was a great place to be. I could exercise and go to the gym and I loved it. Food became something different to before because I was eating so I could exercise properly rather than for the sake of it.

VS, 4 years post surgery
(bypass and revisional surgery)

In the past I've always found dieting easy but keeping the weight off has been the difficult bit. I've been able to do that after bariatric surgery because I can't eat a lot of food – my main meal is on a side plate and I watch what I eat more. It does make you focus on eating healthier stuff. Whereas before my fuel gauge didn't work . . . now it does. Before I could eat a big meal and I'd still feel that I could eat a bit more and a bit more . . . even after a big Christmas dinner I could still pick on chocolates afterwards but now it's completely different. The fuel gauge has re-engaged.

PK, 12 months post bypass

Were the effects of surgery different to what you expected?

I instantly went off food . . . my taste buds changed instantly and I didn't like the taste of sugar at all. It was instant. It was a sudden real-isation that I could only take a few sips of something. It's just realis-ing that you can only eat a tiny amount and feel full straightaway. But I wasn't hungry anyway . . . I was literally eating because I had to.

AE, 18 months post bypass

What are your hopes and reasons for wanting bariatric surgery?

The reasons why people seek surgery are usually a combination of physical, psychological and lifestyle factors. It is a myth that people seek bariatric surgery for mainly appearance reasons.

Physical health reasons for seeking bariatric surgery include wanting to improve diabetes, high blood pressure, pain issues and mobility problems as well as generally improving life expectancy.

The psychological reasons for seeking bariatric surgery include improving confidence, self-esteem and body image as well as wanting to be less anxious about how others may judge them because of their weight. Other reasons include wanting to be more sociable and to form new relationships.

Lifestyle reasons include being less restricted by weight issues and able to engage with more things, to be a more active parent and to be able to return to work.

What are your reasons for wanting bariatric surgery?

What do you hope to get from it?

Is this the right time for you?

It is important to think about the timing of bariatric surgery and as far as possible plan to have it at a time when things in your life are as stable as possible. Sometimes people have stressful things happening in their lives, for example, job uncertainty, caring for a relative or relationship problems, which mean that it is difficult to dedicate enough time to focus on the surgery and everything that goes with it. Although it can be frustrating to delay having the operation, you have just one shot at making this work, so it is important to think about having surgery at a time when you have the greatest chance of making it a success.

Obviously, there are times when unexpected or unpredictable things happen, but are there any potential challenges on the horizon in the following areas?

Relationships and family commitments. Think about your close circle of relationships – your partner (if you have one), family, children – are there any issues that could get in the way of you focusing on surgery? Examples include needing to care for children or relatives, an unsupportive partner, and so on. Who will support and encourage you? Who will support you when you are recovering?

Work. Do you have an erratic work pattern? Do you have regular breaks at work? Is there any risk of redundancy? If you are self-employed, will you be able to financially manage with a period of not working whilst you recover from the surgery?

Finances. Will you have enough money to buy the appropriate foods and supplements? Are there any debt problems causing stress?

Stressful life events. For example, bereavements, relationship difficulties (separations), significant changes in lifestyle, such as a new job, housing issues.

Mental health (see below). Have there been any recent changes in your mental health? Any changes to your medication? Any crisis events?

Other demands on your time. Do you have caring responsibilities? Study commitments?

"I wish they had done an operation on my head as well as my stomach!"

The dramatic weight loss following surgery can also create a different set of psychological adjustments. It is important to think about these as they can impact how you cope with the process and your outcome, both in terms of weight and your psychological wellbeing. Some people find that it's difficult to make the changes that are required for bariatric surgery because they haven't addressed the underlying emotional difficulties or experiences which are driving some of these behaviours in the first place. These are things that surgery does not change.

For those people who have used food as a way of managing emotions or avoiding thinking about difficulties, it can be challenging to have to tolerate and manage these feelings without eating afterwards.

I thought that having bariatric surgery would fix everything . . . I thought it would be a sprinkle of fairy dust and all my problems would go away! Surgery has got rid of my weight issues and that has really helped with my confidence. I can go out and go to places more easily. So it's definitely helped that side of it but it's definitely made me face up to some psychological issues and stop pushing things aside because I don't have food as my coping mechanism anymore.

JT, 9 months post sleeve gastrectomy

It can be difficult for people to accept that the surgery is only a tool and that they will still need to actively work at managing their weight for the rest of their lives.

I don't feel that I've got what I wanted from it completely. I wanted to be slim, to be like everyone else and not have a weight issue. It has been hard not having my expectations met. I suppose there was a bit of a grieving period of realising that I'm never going to be that weight or have that body. When you have weight loss surgery and meet the surgeon you think "I'm giving this problem to you to fix" because that's what I wanted to happen. That's been my biggest learning curve throughout this process . . . it's not a quick fix. It's a lifelong issue and it's never going to go away whether you have weight loss surgery or not, you still have to work at maintaining your weight loss.

NR, bypass, regained weight

What are the psychological risk factors for a poor outcome from surgery?

Some psychological difficulties and behaviours may get in the way of the result that people want from bariatric surgery or affect how they adjust to life after surgery. This does not mean that you are guaranteed to have a poor result if you have these difficulties, but it highlights the importance of being aware of this and to actively work at managing these to reduce the risk.

The research tells us that people who have the following difficulties are at greater risk of having a poor outcome, both in terms of how much weight they lose but also how they feel emotionally. The psychological risk factors that we are aware of are specific eating patterns such as binge eating and emotional eating, grazing and non-adherence to the eating plan. There are also mental health factors such as depression, adjustment difficulties and personality disorders which are associated with poorer weight loss. Having more than one mental health diagnosis (usually personality disorder plus another condition) is associated with poorer weight loss (Kinzl et al. 2006).

Another issue to be mindful of is that some medications used for mental health purposes may need altering after surgery. This is particularly for those people who are considering having a gastric bypass. It is important to make sure that a health professional will monitor and review these medications after surgery.

Being aware of other psychological consequences

There can be unexpected psychological consequences after bariatric surgery that can be complicated to deal with and cope with. For example, whilst it is tempting to assume that rapid weight loss is a cause for celebration, it can be challenging for some people as they struggle to cope with changes in their relationships and other people's reactions to their weight loss. This rapid weight loss can also lead to distorted body image whereby there is a discrepancy between the person logically recognising that they have lost weight but finding it difficult to see this when they look in the mirror. It can also be difficult to anticipate some of the eating challenges that arise, as they are so alien from previous experiences. These may include not feeling hungry and having to push yourself to eat, not enjoying food and so on. Sometimes people are taken by surprise by these reactions and experiences – they have often focused so much on weight loss that they haven't been able to imagine changes or challenges that arise as a result of this.

Excess skin

It can be difficult for people to imagine themselves having a problem or being distressed about excess or loose skin after surgery as they are often so focused on improving their health or things that are of concern to them at that time. As a result of the rapid and large weight loss, excess skin is likely to be an issue for many people, and it can be something which is very upsetting for people to cope with. Sometimes, the distress and dissatisfaction that people have experienced about their weight shifts to distress about the excess skin. Some people would consider having body-contouring surgery, although this can be costly and it is major surgery. Chapter 10 focuses on body image after bariatric surgery and contains more information about this.

Impact on relationships

Some people find that their relationship with their partner or spouse changes after bariatric surgery. It can bring people closer together, but it can also lead to tension and difficulties. This is particularly likely if your partner has weight issues as your lives may start to change and move in different directions. There is some evidence that those who are married or in long-term relationships lose less weight (Ferriby et al. 2015), so it's important to think about the effect of your relationship on your eating behaviour. Does your partner want to make changes? What could get in the way? How does your partner feel about your decision to lose weight?

At this stage, it is helpful to identify your sources of support as well as those people who could sabotage or get in the way of your goals.

Making decisions about who to tell and when

It can be tricky trying to work out who to tell about your plan to have bariatric surgery and when to tell them. It is important to think this through carefully because you can end up being influenced and having to manage other people's reactions and judgements about bariatric surgery. Many people are misinformed about bariatric surgery and think it's either unnecessary, a cheat or a sign of weakness – this has the potential to be very upsetting as well as distracting from your main focus.

My wife simply does not understand why I can't lose weight without having bariatric surgery – she thinks it is just a matter of willpower. She thinks that I should just eat the way that I would need to after surgery and that would solve the problem. She is worried about how other people would view the surgery as she thinks it means I am "giving in" and she is embarrassed about this.

IB, pre bariatric surgery

Relatives and friends may perceive bariatric surgery as being different to other surgical procedures because it is an operation you are choosing to have. This is different to other surgical operations, which we are usually told we *must* have done because they are causing symptoms, for example, having your appendix or gall bladder removed. Relatives and friends may also overestimate the risks of the surgery and perceive it to be very 'risky' – in fact, the death rate following gastric bypass is similar to having your gall bladder removed and lower than following a hip replacement. On the other hand, relatives and friends may be able to provide important support and encouragement through the process.

It can be helpful to arm yourself with accurate and reliable information to give to relatives and friends about bariatric surgery – it is difficult to argue with the evidence about bariatric surgery. For example, 80% of people will go into remission from their diabetes. People generally tend to focus on the risks of having the surgery, but it's equally important to think about the risks of not having the surgery. What is likely to happen to your health and any existing health conditions without the surgery? The research clearly demonstrates that people are much more likely to die from *not* having bariatric surgery. Bariatric surgery significantly reduces the risk of death from heart disease, diabetes and cancer – the diseases strongly associated with obesity. If possible, take relatives to your bariatric appointments so that they can gather information for themselves and have the opportunity to develop confidence in the team.

Although it is obviously preferable to have the support of family and friends, ultimately you may have to make a tough decision about whether to have the surgery regardless. It is not as easy or comfortable if you decide to proceed without their support, but it is still possible.

Summary section

Bariatric surgery can be an incredible opportunity to exit from long-term weight struggles and yo-yo dieting. However, in reality it creates a different set of issues and problems to deal with, although these are usually far more manageable. It is important to develop the insight and skills to manage these emerging challenges in order to get the psychological and weight loss outcome you are hoping for.

References

Courcoulas, A.P. et al., 2013. Weight change and health outcomes at 3 years after bariatric surgery among individuals with severe obesity. *Journal of the American Medical Association*, 15213 (22), 1–10.

Ferriby, M. et al., 2015. Marriage and weight loss surgery: a narrative review of patient and spousal outcomes. *Obesity Surgery*, 25 (12), 2436–2442.

Fildes, A. et al., 2015. Probability of an obese person attaining normal body weight: cohort study using electronic health records. *American Journal of Public Health*, e1–e6.

Kinzl, J.F. et al., 2006. Psychosocial predictors of weight loss after bariatric surgery. *Obesity surgery*, 16 (12), 1609–14.

Ratcliffe, D., Khatun, M., and Ali, R., 2012. Psychological gains and losses following bariatric surgery. *Clinical Psychology Forum*, 239.

Sheets, C.S. et al., 2014. Post-operative psychosocial predictors of outcome in bariatric surgery. *Obesity Surgery*, 25 (2), 330–345.

Chapter 2

Creating new habits and making changes in preparation for bariatric surgery

In this chapter, we will focus on making changes in preparation for bariatric surgery. These changes do not involve going on a "diet" or trying to lose weight right now; the aim is to make sure that you have the behavioural foundations in place to make bariatric surgery work for you. The more effort you put into making changes before surgery, the smoother the transition into post-surgery life.

Your approach to change

You do not have to make lots of changes to your eating all at once. It is better to identify and work on just a couple of changes rather than trying to instigate a completely different system of eating which leads to you becoming overwhelmed and abandoning the plan. At this stage, we are also trying to work on rebuilding your confidence in yourself and your ability to make and embed sustainable changes.

It can also help to try to view any changes that you make as an experiment. This involves keeping an open mind about what the experience and results of the change will be. All that is required is that you make a commitment to test out making a change and then explore how effective it was and how you it made you feel. This approach helps you to step back and make choices based on evidence – this is a powerful place to be!

Much of our eating is habit-based, automatic and out of our awareness

Without truly noticing and recognising your eating patterns, it is difficult to know what changes you need to make to align your behaviour with what is required for surgery. Imagine trying to drive to a new destination in the dark without headlights – it is likely that you would get lost or meet a few obstacles along the way. If you switch the headlights on and use a map, these risks would be reduced dramatically. This information is vital in order to work out what traps you might need to watch out for or issues you might need to work on.

After many years of actively trying to manage your weight through dieting, you may feel that you have good awareness and insight into your eating behaviour. However, we are all creatures of habit and much of what we eat is out of our awareness. In fact, research tells us that people underestimate their calorie intake by approximately 40% (Sarwer et al. 2011). It is not that we are lying or being deceitful: it is simply that we don't notice as our behaviour has become automatic and routine. To put this into context, if you think back over the last week, how many times do you actually remember cleaning your teeth? And how many times were you aware that you were cleaning your teeth at the time that you were brushing them? Or think about a familiar journey that you take most days: are there times that you don't remember travelling to your destination? The first time you pay attention is when you suddenly realise that you have arrived! This is because behaviours that we repeat tend to become habits. We don't pay full attention to these because our brains have implicitly learned to automatically follow a sequence of events.

Why does this happen? One of the reasons that our eating becomes so automatic is that it becomes a type of learned behaviour – this happens when behaviours are repeated many times. Your brain has implicitly learned to recognise that in certain situations, you follow a sequence of behaviours. This means that if you do X, then Y and Z automatically follow. It is a problem of learning too well!

If we learn to follow certain behaviour scripts and pair certain activities together, then we will start to do these automatically without consciously noticing or making an active decision. Common examples of paired eating activities are:

- making a cup of tea and automatically getting a biscuit at the same time
- watching TV and eating snacks at the same time
- coming in at the end of the day and checking the fridge straight away
- drinking beer whilst watching football.

It is helpful to try to disentangle the two behaviours so that you start to unlearn some of the associations you have made. Can you experiment and do one without the other? You will need to be consistent with this so that you form a new habit.

Increasing your awareness of your eating

A food diary will help you to tune in more accurately to your eating behaviour.

There is strong evidence that keeping a food diary is one of the best predictors of weight loss following bariatric surgery. Those people that consistently monitor their eating behaviour are at less risk of regaining weight (Odom et al. 2010). This process of tuning in and evaluating can help you to improve your confidence and sense of control over weight. This awareness of your eating and the choices you make is crucial for life after bariatric surgery – they are foundation skills.

	Morning	Afternoon	Evening
Monday			
Tuesday			
Wednesday			
Thursday			
Friday			
Saturday			
Sunday			

Figure 2.1 Food and drink diary

Diary reflection and planning

What patterns do you notice in your diary?

What do you need to focus on next?

You can also choose what you want to record in your diary. A basic food diary is included, which you can modify to fit your circumstances.

If you instinctively feel that you want to avoid keeping a food diary, try to identify the reasons or the thoughts behind this – are you prepared to consider trying one as an experiment? What do you have to lose?

Common blocks to completing a food diary

Worries about being judged. Sometimes people worry that health-care professionals will judge their food diary like a homework assignment. This can lead people to avoid doing them or creating an "edited" version of their eating patterns where they just write the "good" foods. It's important to be clear that the purpose of doing the food diary is for you and only you. Think about what would be helpful for you to know – you don't have to share these with anyone unless you would find it helpful. You have complete control over what you record and how you do it.

Being confronted by reality. Sometimes people are apprehensive about keeping a food diary because writing it down somehow makes it more real. Some people feel very ashamed and embarrassed about their eating patterns so seeing this written down can feel painful and exposing. Shame often leads to people trying to conceal or hide their eating. This is a very obvious thing to say, but just because it isn't written down, it doesn't mean it didn't happen. Whilst the diary may feel difficult to do at first, it will get easier, and these feelings of shame will fade. You can even just try it for one day at a time and build up to doing it more consistently. Even imagining yourself writing down what you are eating is a helpful first step towards actually doing it. Keeping a diary is a sign of your commitment to change and demonstrates a willingness to be honest and truthful with yourself – give yourself credit for this.

What's the point? I know what I eat. It is worth double-checking that belief to make sure it is accurate. Of course, you may be absolutely correct that you do know exactly what you eat – in which case, it would be good to be reassured about that. However, the evidence consistently suggests that most people underestimate their food intake by at least 40% because of their automatic eating patterns.

Finding time and/or remembering to do the diary. There are different ways of keeping a food diary. These include:

- using an online food tracking app
- making notes on your mobile phone of what you have eaten
- having a specific notepad to keep your food diary
- emailing yourself
- taking photos of what you have eaten.

Strategies that will remind you to update your diary include coinciding doing your diary with another activity so you have a behavioural anchor, for example, whenever you make a cup of tea or visit the bathroom. You may also find it helpful to ask someone else to remind you. Other people find it helpful to set an alarm on their phone as a prompt.

When reviewing your food diary, it's important to get a balance between identifying some problem areas as well as identifying what you are doing well. This will help you to get into a balanced mindset of looking for the positives and negatives, not just focusing on what you are doing "wrong". This sort of balanced approach can help with maintaining motivation and help you feel less overwhelmed.

Getting into a regular eating pattern

It is very common for people who struggle with their weight to have an irregular eating pattern. The most common pattern involves skipping breakfast and lunch (or eating just very small amounts during the day) and having a large meal in the evening. Most people have been on diets that have involved restricting the number of calories, so they often think that skipping meals will lead to weight loss. Furthermore, it may seem illogical to eat regularly, as the assumption is that this will lead to weight gain. We are often told that eating regularly is important, yet the reasons for this are often not clear.

What does the evidence tell us?

Research published by Masheb and Grilo (2006) looked at the number of meals and snacks eaten by people whose weight placed them in the obese category. They found that nearly half of these people skipped breakfast. Those people who ate breakfast every day weighed less than those who didn't eat breakfast. Also, those people who ate three meals per day weighed less than those who skipped meals. Of the three meals per day, breakfast appears to be the most important in being related to lower weight. There is other compelling evidence for starting to eat breakfast from the National Weight Control Registry. This registry has followed up people who have successfully maintained weight loss in order to identify what it is that they do that helps them keep their weight off. It appears that eating breakfast is one of those important factors. Very few people (less than 5%) who have successfully maintained weight loss skip breakfast (Wyatt et al. 2002). Skipping breakfast is very uncommon amongst those who have been able to lose weight and maintain this weight loss. This challenges the idea that skipping breakfast helps with weight loss.

What happens when you skip meals?

Many studies show that when people skip meals or have periods of fasting, they then tend to lose control of their eating and eat larger amounts. This is because hunger builds during the day, and when people skip meals, they go into "starvation mode". This is not related to someone's weight: it refers to how someone's body responds if they have not eaten. As a result of restricting their energy supply (i.e. food), binge eating is the body's way of trying to correct this energy deficit. The body starts to send strong signals that food is needed to preserve and protect it – the body has an increasingly urgent need for energy. This is the point at which people often start to experience cravings for high sugar foods and when overeating or binge eating is likely to kick in. When people haven't eaten for many hours, it also affects the way the brain works – it affects the part of the brain that makes decisions, and people are more likely to make impulsive decisions.

Hopefully, you can now see why it is important to start getting into the habit of eating regularly, especially as it is a very important aspect of the post-surgery eating plan. After surgery, you may not necessarily feel hungry, and this can lead to skipping meals, which in turn can lead to poor health and malnutrition. Also, because the stomach is much smaller after surgery, people are not able to make up for meals they miss earlier in the day by having a large meal later. One of the major benefits of eating regularly is that it can really help to regulate and manage your mood, particularly if you are prone to mood swings. It can also help with feelings of tiredness. Many people find that by starting to eat regularly, their emotional eating or binge eating reduces dramatically.

Strategies to eat more regularly

It may take time and persistence to get used to eating regularly, as it may feel alien and "wrong" at first, but stick with it; it will get easier, and you will see the benefits.

Question your thinking and decision-making. We often have different expectations and ideas about what is an acceptable way to treat ourselves versus what we consider acceptable for other people. For example, would you allow your children (or loved ones) to go out in the morning without food and not eat again until the end of the day when they get home? I'm sure that none of you would allow or want this to happen, so why would you treat yourself in that way?

Resetting your "stomach clock". You need to eat regularly for a rea-sonable period of time (at least a month) in order to feel the effects. Most people find that it can take a while to re-educate the body so that it learns to expect food at a certain time. It takes a while to reset our internal body clock. For example, you may automatically wake up at a set time when you have to go to work because you have repeated this over a period of time. Along similar lines, your stomach will start to expect food at a certain time if you start to eat regularly. Some peo-ple find it helpful to work out set time points to eat (you can set an alarm as a further prompt). Everyone's day starts and ends at dif-ferent times, so you have to work out a way of eating three regular meals that fit within your routine. It's useful to just try eating regularly and see what happens – that way you can at least make an informed decision about what the advantages and disadvantages are for you.

Planning ahead. Some people find it helpful to go a step further and start to use a meal-planning diary that they fill out in advance. This is a really positive option which involves you using your "thinking brain" to do your decision-making and planning ahead for your eating. It can also help you to avoid making impulsive choices based on what is easily available to you at the time that you need to eat. You've already done the thinking work ahead of time, so this gives you a really good safety net to prevent you going off track. You can use the meal plan to form a shopping list for the week.

Updating and challenging subconscious childhood rules about eating

Much of our learning about our eating comes from our early childhood and family experiences and the eating environment that we grew up in. Many of the rules that we were taught as children are implicit. We are not fully aware of these rules, but they are operating in the background, guiding and driving our behaviour. For example:

> When I was growing up we were encouraged to eat as much as we could as quickly as possible – in fact my mother used to shout "champion!" to whoever finished first. It means that I still eat very quickly and find it difficult to slow down my eating now.
>
> AE, 18 months post bypass

Some common examples of these early eating rules include:

> You have to eat everything on your plate.
> You must not leave anything.
> If you don't eat your food quickly then someone else will eat it.
> If you don't eat your main course then you can't have pudding.

Spend a few minutes thinking back to your mealtimes and what your eating behaviour was like as a child.

- What happened if you left food?
- What happened if you didn't like a particular food?
- Were you given food as a treat or reward?
- Were there any issues with food not being available or restricted?
- What did you learn as a result of these experiences?
- How does this affect your eating behaviour in the here and now?

These early eating rules and behaviours develop for reasons that make complete sense at the time – the problem is that we continue to behave in the same way, even though we are no longer in the same situation. We need to work at updating our memories and the information we have about the possible consequences of sticking to or breaking these early eating rules.

For example, what happens if you leave food? If you don't eat quickly, will someone else steal your food? Try to identify the unhelpful childhood rules that guide your eating behaviour and experiment with breaking them to find out what happens.

Finding the "had enough" point – the hunger and fullness scale

People often think of themselves as being either hungry *or* full – this can create problems. Over time, some people may have started to believe that if they are not full, then it must mean they are hungry – this sets them up for a grazing pattern where they keep topping up on food to avoid feeling hungry. Some people are worried or frightened by the thought of feeling hungry and so actively try to avoid this feeling by overeating. Feelings of anxiety and hunger can feel quite similar (e.g. "butterflies" in the stomach) so some people confuse these.

People's perception of fullness changes over time as portion sizes increase, so this can lead to needing to eat more food before feeling full. Our feelings of fullness become skewed over time, and we start to redefine what it means for us to feel full. It is helpful to think of hunger and fullness as being on a rating scale with degrees of hunger and fullness in between the extremes. The next exercise is about helping you tune into how hungry and full you feel after eating and investigating the middle ground between hungry and feeling full.

- Think about how hungry you feel before eating.
- How full do you feel after eating?
- Where do you think you should be on the hunger and fullness scale before and after eating?
- Can you imagine what it would feel like to experience 7/10 fullness?
- Can you tell the difference between feeling full, not feeling hungry and feeling satisfied? What are the different ratings associated with these?
- What point are you on the scale when you actively decide to have your last mouthful of food?

One man who had the belief that "if he wasn't extremely full, then he was hungry" used the hunger/fullness rating scale before and after he had eaten. This helped him to tune into some of the sensations along the

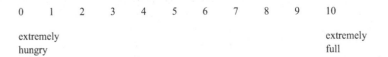

Figure 2.2 Hunger and fullness scale

rating scale and to recognise that there were degrees of fullness, rather than just an extreme version of fullness.

Mindful eating and creating vivid food memories

It is now time to switch our attention to *how* you eat. Mindful eating involves paying full attention to the process of eating and activating all your senses to notice the appearance, taste, smell, temperature and texture of food.

This process of tuning in to how we eat is important to life after bariatric surgery, when it is really important to get the maximum enjoyment out of small amounts of food.

Mindful eating exercise

For this exercise, you will need one of the following – a raisin, a grape, a cherry tomato, a strawberry etc. You will need to do this in a quiet place with no distractions.

Before you start the exercise, rate on a scale of 1–10 how hungry you feel. Where do you zoom into in your body to notice hunger?

Imagine that you are an alien landed on Earth, and that you have never seen this particular food item before – you have no idea what its texture is, how it may taste and whether you may like it or not.

First, look at the food you have chosen. Look at its colour, shape and surface texture. What do you notice about it?

Now bring the food up to your nose and gently sniff it – can you detect any smell? Is it sweet or savoury? Does it feel hot, cold or room temperature?

Now gently place the food into your mouth but *do not bite it.* Just allow it to be in your mouth – roll the food around and explore it with your tongue. What do you notice? How does it feel?

Now take a bite. After biting it, roll it around again in your mouth and explore it with your tongue. What do you notice now that you have taken a bite? How has the texture changed? And the taste?

Now chew the food and notice the changes in texture and taste. What sensations do you notice? You may notice the urge to swallow the food – try to resist this for a while and just notice what it feels like.

When you decide to swallow the food, pay attention and try to track the food as it leaves your mouth and goes down into your stomach.

As you finish this exercise, re-rate your hunger on a scale of 1–10 – has it changed?

It takes time to become familiar with these mindful eating exercises, so don't worry if you find them difficult or feel silly trying them. The process of slowing down and paying full attention to each aspect and part of the eating process sometimes leads people to discover that they don't actually like the foods that they previously thought they enjoyed eating! By paying more attention to your eating, you will create a more vivid memory about the food that you have eaten. Evidence shows that this helps people feel satisfied and full for longer, and that they are less likely to want to continue eating. Researchers have found that by enhancing people's memories of what they have eaten recently (just by simply asking them to recall what they have eaten), their meal sizes go down later in the day (Higgs 2005).

Another consequence of slowing down is that it can help you to notice and recognise different degrees of hunger and fullness, so that you get a better sense of where you are on the scale.

Thinking traps that affect your eating behaviour

Various thinking patterns affect our eating choices and decisions. Sometimes we are very conscious of these thoughts as they are very dominant and noisy; for example, there are times when it can feel as though there is an argument going on in our minds, usually along the lines of "I want X" versus "You can't have X". It is helpful to identify these thoughts as they guide and influence our behaviour.

If we can rewind to identify any thoughts driving our eating behaviour then the behaviour starts to make more sense. We often tend to focus on our behaviour as the problem, but it is often our thoughts that drive our behaviour so we need to target these. Our thoughts are the spark that lights the flame. There's always a thought process behind a behaviour, even though we may not necessarily be conscious of it.

Thoughts ———————————▶ Behaviour

Common thinking habits and patterns that may influence your eating

Thought pattern	Behaviour
Permission-giving thoughts E.g. "Oh, go on, I deserve a treat".	Abandon plan and eat "forbidden" foods.
Can't be bothered thoughts E.g. "It's too much hassle".	Pick convenience options.
Pessimistic thoughts E.g. "It's not going to work/ There's no way I can do it".	Don't engage with making a plan.
Emotional eating thoughts E.g. "Eating X will make me feel better".	Eat extra high-calorie foods that aren't part of the eating plan.
Perfectionistic thoughts E.g. "I have to change my eating completely and stick to the plan 100%".	Get overwhelmed with changes and find it hard to get back on track when a setback is experienced.
Intrusive thoughts about food E.g. "I want X (food) . . . No, you can't have it because X isn't part of your plan . . . I want X . . .".	Easier to give in and eat than have to tolerate and manage these intrusive thoughts. This is a thought management problem, not a food problem.

Figure 2.3 How do thought patterns impact our eating behaviour?

How can you start to identify your thoughts?

The first thing is to turn up the volume of these thoughts so that we can become more aware of them. That also means that we can make more active decisions about whether they are helping or hindering us.

Think about the last time that you made an eating choice that you were unhappy with. Now try to rewind the clock to try to work out what led to that choice.

Where were you? What was happening? How were you feeling?

If we could rewind and turn the volume up to hear your internal conversation and what you were saying to yourself, what would we have heard you saying?

Did your thoughts fall into any of the categories listed above?

What was the outcome of having that thought – how did it affect your eating?

It is possible to step back and challenge these thoughts so that they have less impact on our eating or ability to stick to the eating plan. Figure 2.4 shows some alternative ways of stepping back and responding to the thoughts that create problems with our eating or weight. If you refer back to the thinking patterns that you previously identified as problematic, can you start to create some alternative thoughts to challenge and counteract these? You may want to use some of the ones listed below or you may want to create your own.

Thought pattern	Alternative thoughts
Permission-giving thoughts E.g. "Oh, go on, I deserve a treat".	There are different ways of treating myself other than through food.
Can't be bothered thoughts E.g. "It's too much hassle".	It might take more effort in the short term but I will feel good about making the effort later. And at least I won't feel guilty and bad about what I chose to eat.
Pessimistic thoughts E.g. "It's not going to work/ There's no way I can do it".	I could give it a try and then decide whether it's worth doing after collecting some evidence and then deciding.
Emotional eating thoughts E.g. "Eating X will make me feel better".	There are other ways of making myself feel better. Food has just become my default but there are other options (see Chapter 3).
Perfectionistic thoughts E.g. "I have to change my eating completely and stick to the plan 100%".	When I try these extreme options its difficult to keep going. Although it feels odd – I need to focus on making changes step by step.
Intrusive thoughts about food E.g. "I want X (food) . . . No, you can't have it because X isn't part of your plan . . . I want X . . .".	These are just thoughts – they will come and go. I need to find something else to focus on.

Figure 2.4 Recognising and managing problematic thought patterns

Changing your food environment – practical strategies

Sometimes it is easier to change your environment rather than think about changing yourself! It's about making sure that you set things up in a way that makes it easier to behave in ways that fit with your weight loss goal. A good example of this is when people stop keeping the foods that tempt them at home.

Plates and portion sizes

Think about how you serve food – what do you serve it in? What size are your plates?

Research tells us that when food is served on larger plates, people will generally eat much more. A psychologist, Brian Wansink, compared the amount of soup that two groups of people ate and how full they felt after eating it. However, there was a twist to the study. One group had a normal bowl of soup and the other group had soup from bottomless bowls that were constantly being topped up by a secret pipe underneath. He found that people who had the bottomless, constantly refilling bowls ate 73% more, yet they did not rate themselves as being fuller than those who just had the normal bowls. This demonstrates that we tend to eat with our eyes and rely on visual cues rather than sensations of fullness from our stomach. The more food there is, the more we eat. This is why it is so important to be careful about your portion sizes and the type of plates you use.

Strategies

Experiment with using smaller plates. This is good practice for after surgery when you will need to use much smaller plates and bowls for your meals because your portion sizes will reduce. These small plates and bowls can be a useful way of setting limits and giving feedback about whether you are on track.

Another way of reducing your portion sizes is to change the proportions of food groups on your plate. Aim for half of your plate to be vegetables or salad, one quarter protein and one quarter carbohydrates.

Food shopping

You may need to consider changing the way you do your food shopping. It helps to proactively think and plan how you buy and shop for food.

Obviously, food shops go out of their way to tempt us with special offers and bakery smells. Be careful of special offers and reduced items: they may seem like a bargain at the time but do they fit with your goals? It is possible to create a positive chain reaction. If you plan your eating in advance and then shop for foods that are consistent with this plan, you are much more likely to eat those foods because they will be easily available.

One of the challenges people sometimes experience is managing their eating plan alongside others who may not be following the same plan. For example, if your partner is not trying to lose weight and still wants to have treats like chocolate and crisps at home, how will you manage this? It is important to talk about it so that you agree a plan. There are some practical ideas that might help, such as keeping their treats somewhere else (e.g. having their own cupboard, leaving them in their car) or only eating those foods outside the home.

Potential strategies

- It may sound obvious, but try writing a shopping list ... and stick to it! Set yourself the rule that if there is something extra you are tempted by, then you must leave the shop without buying it and go back to buy it separately. This will give your brain a bit of time to catch up. It is surprising how often the extra effort puts people off!
- Review your shopping list – is it consistent with your plan and goals?
- Try shopping online. Some people find this more helpful as it avoids the temptation of walking up and down the different shopping aisles. You can also set up a regular food order.
- Work out a menu plan (you can decide how far in advance you want to plan) and work out your shopping list based on this plan.
- Talk to your family about how you/they will manage treats in the home.

Introducing the golden rules for eating after surgery

There are some specific eating guidelines you will need to follow after surgery focused on **how** you eat. They are important because they will help you avoid pain, regurgitation after eating and help you maintain your weight loss. It can take time to get used to some of these new eating behaviours as they may seem unfamiliar and unnatural, so it is advisable to start practising these before your operation.

The "golden rules" for eating after bariatric surgery are:

- Take bites no bigger than the size of your thumbnail – it can help to use a teaspoon or children's cutlery when eating.
- Chew at least 20 times or until your food is the consistency of puree before swallowing.
- Wait between bites and put your cutlery down (you should aim for one bite per minute).
- Stop eating after about 20 minutes.
- Avoid drinking and eating at the same time. Don't drink for 10 minutes before eating and then wait for 30 minutes after eating. This will help avoid overfilling your stomach pouch and regurgitating. If you eat and drink at the same time after surgery, this means you will flush food through your stomach, which means you are less likely to feel full, and it can therefore trigger hunger.
- Sit down to eat – this will help you to avoid getting into a habit of grazing.

Other habits that need to be addressed before bariatric surgery

Most people are aware that they will need to make changes to their eating behaviour as part of bariatric surgery, but some other lifestyle habits may also need to be addressed. It is important to be aware of these so that you can start to address one thing at a time rather than trying to change everything all at once.

Smoking

It is important to stop smoking before surgery. Some services will require you to stop smoking six months before and the absolute minimum requirement is six weeks. Smoking is problematic after surgery because it is associated with increased rates of complications (including death), it prolongs healing and there is an increased risk of infection. Furthermore, there is an increased risk of developing ulcers at the connection point between the stomach pouch and the intestines. Most people have bariatric surgery to improve their health, and therefore stopping smoking is also an important part of this. It is easy to access help and support to quit smoking through a smoking cessation service.

Alcohol

It is recommended that people abstain from alcohol after bariatric surgery (particularly if you have a bypass). This is because alcohol is absorbed differently and remains in the system for longer – which means that people become intoxicated much faster from a small amount of alcohol. Research consistently shows that there is an increased risk of alcohol dependency after having a gastric bypass, so it is better to abstain. For those people who have a history of alcohol dependency or heavy habitual use of alcohol, most services will require you to be abstinent from alcohol for 12 months prior to surgery (and may recommend not having gastric bypass surgery). The other reason for avoiding alcohol after surgery is the empty calories it contains.

Summary

Now is the time to start making some changes to the way you manage your eating. The aim is to make these changes so that you are slowly adjusting your habits and behaviour so that the transition to life after surgery is as smooth as possible.

References

Higgs, S., 2005. Memory and its role in appetite regulation. *Physiology and Behavior*, 85 (1), 67–72.

Masheb, R.M. and Grilo, C.M., 2006. Eating patterns and breakfast consumption in obese patients with binge eating disorder. *Behaviour Research and Therapy*, 44 (11), 1545–53.

Odom, J., et al. 2010. Behavioral predictors of weight regain after bariatric surgery. *Obesity Surgery*, 20 (3), 349–356.

Sarwer, D.B., et al. 2011. Dietary intake and eating behaviour after bariatric surgery: threats to weight loss maintenance and strategies for success. *Surgery for Obesity & Related Diseases*, 7, 644–651.

Wyatt, H.R. et al., 2002. Long-term weight loss and breakfast in subjects in the National Weight Control Registry. *Obesity Research*, 10 (2), 78–82.

Chapter 3

Understanding and managing your emotional relationship with food

In this chapter, we will focus on eating which is related to how you are feeling emotionally and not driven by physical hunger. Being physically hungry is only one reason why we choose to eat; many different things can influence our eating choices and behaviour. Our emotions and our moods are major influences on our eating behaviours.

Eating in response to emotions is something that affects most people (whether overweight or not), but it can become problematic if it becomes a regular pattern and becomes one of your main ways of coping. There are a range of emotions and moods that can affect our eating, including sadness, stress, boredom, happiness, anxiety, anger and so on. In the first part of the chapter, we will focus on identifying the extent to which emotional eating is an issue for you and developing an understanding of how and why this has become a problem. The final part of the chapter focuses on some of the strategies that you can start to introduce. It might be tempting to fast forward to the section about strategies in the hope of finding a "fix", but in order to find a strategy that will work, you need to spend time understanding the problem.

Our emotional connections with food start to form and develop from an early age and are often an accepted part of our culture – for example, birthdays are celebrated with cake, and Christmas is associated with overindulging in certain foods or large meals. In addition, we are often encouraged to think about food as an emotional tonic or something that can enhance our mood or take away negative feelings by advertisers. Examples of this include Mars' Celebrations chocolates and McDonald's Happy Meals.

These emotional connections with food become problematic when eating becomes our main way of coping with situations that affect us emotionally. It is important to develop ways of managing emotional eating alongside bariatric surgery for a few reasons:

- Bariatric surgery does not change your emotional responses or the life challenges that may lead you to feel certain emotions.
- Research tells us that those people who have a pattern of emotional eating are at risk of losing less weight after bariatric surgery (White et al. 2010; Scholtz et al. 2007).
- Most people who have this pattern of eating describe feeling unhappy about it as it tends to lead to feelings of guilt and feeling out of control. These feelings in turn can perpetuate emotional eating.

Emotional eating is a very common problem amongst people seeking bariatric surgery. Research from our bariatric surgery service has found that 60% of people attending an assessment appointment before bariatric surgery reported emotional eating patterns. In fact, many people also feel that their emotional eating is a factor that has contributed to their weight problems or made it difficult for them to lose weight. When we ask people what factors they think have caused or contributed to their weight problems, emotional eating comes out as the most common reason.

Below are some quotes from people describing their emotional eating patterns before surgery.

Food was my solution for everything . . . happy, sad, anything that was going on in my life. It was soothing and calming to eat after an emotional upset or when my feelings were hurt. Food would never hurt me like people did . . . it would never let me down or argue with me. But realistically it does hurt you in the end because you keep gaining weight but it is difficult to know how to break out of this pattern.

SB, 3 years post surgery

I never had a meal plan . . . I never had any sort of structure for my eating and I just picked throughout the day. I never kept an eye on what I was eating or how much. If I was depressed I could go through packets and packets of biscuits. I would eat to make myself feel ill. It used to stop me thinking. If I got depressed or upset, food was there . . . it was a comfort in some ways. I wouldn't eat to make me happy, I would eat until I was ill or sore. In some ways it used to make me feel better to feel so bad after eating.

ST, 2.5 years post sleeve gastrectomy

The vicious cycle of emotional eating

The vicious cycle of emotional eating occurs when people eat in response to certain emotions, often in an attempt to make themselves feel better. Whilst this type of eating does often make people feel better in the short term, this tends to be transient. These feelings tend to be quickly replaced with feelings of guilt, shame and regret about eating.

This cycle is problematic for a couple of reasons. First, it can have a damaging effect on someone's self-esteem because they feel ashamed and guilty at the same time as feeling powerless to stop the cycle. It can also be very difficult and frustrating for people to understand why they are behaving in a way that is the direct opposite of their intentions and goals. Second, it can mean that people become more and more dependent on food as a way of coping in order to get that short-term mood boost – it can almost become a bit of an addictive cycle.

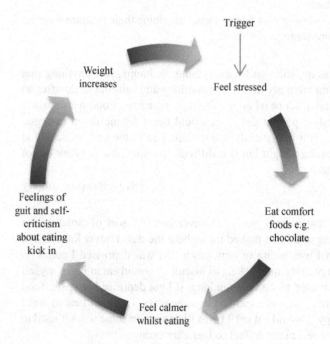

Figure 3.1 Vicious cycle of emotional eating

I hated my eating and I hated food. I felt that I couldn't stop and that I had no control. Food controlled me, not the other way round. There was lots of binge eating and guilt about the binge eating. I needed food but I hated it. When I was binge eating it would get rid of anxiety and any other negative emotions I was feeling but then a few minutes later that feeling would be gone and you would be just left with the guilt and think "Why did I do that? I'm just going to get fatter now".

JT, 9 months post sleeve gastrectomy

We generally do things and repeat them because they work for us on some level – this is also the case with emotional eating. There is a function and purpose to the behaviour. Or rather, it used to have a function and purpose at some point earlier in our lives. We believe that eating makes us feel better, lifts our mood, calms us or stops us feeling bored. However, those benefits tend to be short-lived, and we often feel guilty or ashamed about this pattern of eating or that we have gone off track with the eating plan and that our weight has increased. The balance between the benefits and costs of this pattern of eating starts to tilt in the wrong direction. Whilst at one time, there may have been lots of benefits, this changes over time and it can become something that makes us unhappy and that makes us feel out of control. Stopping to question and evaluate whether these emotional eating patterns do actually fulfil the intended purpose of making us feel better (or less bad) can be the start of updating the beliefs that drive the behaviour.

The quote below is from a woman who was addressing her strong patterns of emotional eating before surgery. It became clear that these patterns of eating served a purpose earlier in her life but no longer worked for her in the here and now. The paragraph below is something that we developed together in an appointment and was something that she would frequently refer to when she felt the urge to emotionally eat.

When I was a child, I developed the belief that eating food was a way of calming myself down when I was feeling very emotional – this worked for me at that time as my mum didn't show me affection. I was independent from an early age and eating played a role in this. It helped me manage how I was feeling and it helped me at the time. However, these old eating strategies no longer work for me now as my weight goes up and I feel unhappy.

MJ, pre surgery

Often, people may have lost sight of the emotional need that they are trying to fulfil with food. Sometimes this is because the emotional connection with eating is often formed early in life when we don't necessarily have the language to express ourselves verbally. We just learn that food makes us feel better! There is an implicit physical and emotional memory that eating is something that helps when we are feeling a particular way. It can be a deep-rooted pattern for those people who experienced difficult experiences earlier in their life – for example, abuse (physical, sexual or emotional) or witnessing violence at home – and where food became connected with making them feel temporarily better or safe. We usually don't question why we react to events in certain ways, and this is particularly the case for patterns of behaviour that are longstanding.

An emotional eating pattern is often just a sticking plaster as it doesn't actually address the situation or problem that led to the emotion or even deal with the feelings effectively. This pattern of eating means that we end up with double the problems – the problem or difficulty that originally triggered the emotional eating, and then on top of that, the additional problem of shame about this pattern of eating and weight gain.

How much do your emotions affect your eating?

It can sometimes be difficult to work out whether you are eating in response to physical hunger (stomach hunger) or hunger that is driven by emotions (head hunger). Obviously, the strategies to deal with these are quite different! Figure 3.2 highlights some of the key differences between stomach and head hunger – these are just a starting point as you will have your own unique experiences to add.

Stomach hunger	Head hunger
Large gap between meals	Connected with emotional state
Rumbling stomach/feel lightheaded	Crave specific foods
Feeling of emptiness in stomach	Thoughts about food
Eating leads to satiety	Eating does not necessarily lead to feeling satisfied or less hungry

Figure 3.2 Differences between stomach hunger and head hunger

Head hunger tends to be a response to certain emotional states which trigger a thought process about wanting (craving) certain foods, whereas stomach hunger is about physical feelings and is usually a prompt that you haven't eaten or that it is time to eat.

Just knowing that there is a difference between these types of hunger can prompt you to start questioning which you may be experiencing at the time. Simply asking, "Where is this urge to eat coming from – my head or stomach?" is a good starting point. It helps you to step back from your automatic responses. It also makes it more likely that if you can work out which type of hunger you are experiencing, then you may be able to use more appropriate strategies to manage it.

Which emotions affect your eating?

In the next section, we will start to identify some of the emotional triggers which affect your eating. Sometimes we assume that emotional eating is always triggered by negative emotions such as stress or sadness, but it can happen in response to any emotion. Our emotions are on a spectrum ranging from negative to neutral to positive – all these emotions can potentially affect eating behaviour, but we will each have our own unique emotional triggers along this spectrum. Some people will find that their eating is more influenced by negative emotions, whereas for others, neutral emotions such as boredom are more influential.

Stress		Happiness
Sadness	Boredom	Excited
Anger		Relieved

Look at the following list of emotions – which of these do you think most affect your eating behaviour? There are often a few that jump off the page! This list is just a starting point; there may be other emotions that aren't on the list that affect your eating.

If you can learn to recognise and name specific emotions that affect your eating, you can start to spot these emotions at an earlier stage and recognise them for what they are (i.e. emotions) before responding to them through eating. This process of recognition and labelling can help you gain some distance.

Once you have worked out what particular emotions affect your eating, we need to rewind and identify what led to those emotions being

Excited	Loved	Irritated	Nervous	Hurt
Bored	Disappointed	Annoyed	Worried	Ashamed
Happy	Angry	Anxious	Stressed	Guilty
Content	Relieved	Scared	Overwhelmed	Down
Panicked	Helpless	Sad	Embarrassed	Lonely

Figure 3.3 Which emotions affect your eating?

triggered. One of the best ways of doing this is through keeping an emotional eating diary to increase your awareness and help you track your emotional eating triggers and patterns. The diary is a helpful way of rewinding and breaking down the process of emotional eating – it helps you identify the triggers for the emotions, the type of emotions experienced, how these affected your eating and how you felt afterwards.

When you have kept the diary for a while, you can use the information to help you identify:

• how frequently you emotionally eat
• whether there are particular places where it is more likely to occur
• whether there are particular triggers – either emotions or events
• particular foods that you tend to eat
• how you tend to feel afterwards.

All this information is incredibly valuable because it will help you to develop awareness and understanding. This means that rather than being

Day/time/ location	Trigger – what happened to affect your mood?	What emotions were you experiencing? E.g. stress, anxiety, depression, happiness	What thoughts went through your mind that led to eating? E.g. "What the hell"/"Don't care"	What did you eat?	What did you think and feel afterwards?

Figure 3.4 Emotional eating diary

trapped and stuck in the vicious cycle of emotional eating, you start to recognise the pattern from the outside.

It is important to actively look for times when we don't respond to emotional triggers in the same way – these provide valuable information and answers. For example, if you have a pattern of eating in response to stress and find that this happens on 80% of the occasions when you are stressed, what is happening on the other 20% of occasions? Finding out what is happening when there are exceptions to the usual pattern is just as important as understanding the pattern itself. We naturally tend to pay more attention to when things don't go according to plan and the mistakes that we make – this means that we often overlook the times when we behave differently. If we can figure out what is different when we don't emotionally eat in response to our usual triggers, we are a few steps ahead!

How does emotional eating develop?

Much of our learning about eating and how to manage emotions happens early in life. For example, imagine a child who is given sweets by their parents when they are upset (to stop them crying). If this scenario is repeated over time, the brain will learn to make a connection between being upset and having sweets. The brain draws the conclusion based on this learning that "upsetting emotions change or become less difficult when you eat sweets". Once this implicit learning has been cemented, then a template is set which is ready to be activated next time a difficult emotion arises. It makes perfect logical sense that someone would then eat in response to upsetting or difficult emotions because they have learned through experience that eating helps to change that emotion.

The quotes below are examples of the type of emotional connections that people have made with food because of the circumstances and situation that they were in.

I didn't have the best of family homes growing up. When I went to my grandparents, they spoiled me and my sister by giving us cakes and sweets. I felt safe at my grandparents. When we went there with my parents, it's the only place that my father was nice. It was a safe place to be. I think eating and food became connected with that safe feeling. I moved to London for a job and it was so stressful and difficult. When I used to get home at the end of the day, the first thing I would do is eat . . . it helped relieve stress. It would help me calm down. I would go out to work and I had some friends but I didn't like going out. I put this mask on all day to hide how stressed and anxious I was but once I got home back to safety I would just start eating again.

ST, 2.5 years post sleeve gastrectomy

I learned to comfort eat from an early age. I come from a very violent and dysfunctional background and there were always people around me who would say "Oh never mind, here's a bar of chocolate". My grandparents were always giving me food to compensate for my father's behaviour – that was their answer because there wasn't money. Even when I fell over as a child, instead of being given a plaster, I was given a biscuit. And then you start to associate "When I feel bad, I feel better because I've had a bar of chocolate" and you now get to my age of 60 and it's a difficult habit to break.

SB, 3 years post surgery

My mum put me on a diet from when I was about four. Food in our house was the cure-all . . . you fell over, you got fed . . . you didn't fall over, you got fed. My mother used to put loads of butter on the bread and that's a real problem food for me now. I try to avoid it now because I used to coat everything in butter for no good reason but it's so deep-seated that it's a comfort for me.

VS, 4 years post surgery (bypass and revisional)

I absolutely loved food as a child. I can remember being four and my mum worked in a shop and sometimes I would have to go with her. I was demanding and she wanted me to be quiet so she gave me food I liked to keep me quiet. The more weight I put on, the more I ate. By the time I was 8 I was on a diet.

GM, 3.5 years post bypass

As you can see from these quotes, eating is often associated with providing comfort and making difficult things better and more bearable in early childhood. These patterns continue into adulthood and can feel difficult to break because they have become familiar and automatic. Most children do not experience guilt, regret or shame about this pattern of eating – it is only later in life when people become concerned about managing their weight that these problems kick in. This is because on the one hand, people are often actively trying to manage their weight through dieting, but then on the other hand, they are trying to manage their emotions through old patterns of eating. It is often a hard balance to strike.

As you can see, food can become very deeply connected with early memories so that we start to associate the specific food itself with a feeling of being cared for, loved, nurtured, protected and so on. This is one of the reasons why people may crave or want specific foods when they are feeling emotional – sometimes it is possible to trace back to discover that these foods have a certain meaning or emotional feeling attached to them.

When I was little my mum always used to make me a sugar sandwich when I was upset or something had gone wrong. I still have
sugar sandwiches now when I am upset.

WL, pre surgery

One woman experienced strong cravings for a particular type of childhood
sweet when feeling anxious. When she ate these sweets, she associated
them with feeling safe and relieved. It was difficult for her to understand
why she always craved these sweets when she was feeling anxious until
we traced back the connections she had with them. As a child, she had
been sexually abused and was given these particular sweets after each
episode of abuse ended. She had learned to associate the feeling of safety
and relief that the abuse had ended with eating these sweets. These emotional connections with food usually start to make sense when we trace
back to find out more about where and how those connections were made.

Let's now turn to think about whether any of your early experiences
are connected with your eating behaviour and what associations you may
have developed and learned as a result. The aim is to try to look for connections and see whether they are unknowingly impacting your eating in
the here and now.

Past experiences, food and mood connections

Some of the common associations with food that people may have made
earlier in life are listed below. Do these apply to you?

You can now start to join up and make connections between the col-
umns in Figure 3.5, for example:

If I feel X (emotion) then I eat Y and this makes me feel Z (emotion).

If I feel upset, then I eat sweets and this makes me feel calmer.

What connections and beliefs can you identify?

Many people find that breaking it down in this way and making these
links really helps them to understand the context and reasons for why they
may eat in this way. Connections from the past may be remembered and
things that didn't necessarily make sense before start to fall into place.

How do these connections fit in? If you look at the vicious cycle of
emotional eating in Figure 3.6, these beliefs usually bridge the connection between mood and food and drive our behaviour.

Some people have problems with emotional eating later in life because
they were deprived of food as a child. They may not have had access to

If you were:	Did you eat in these situations?	What foods would you have?
Upset		
Well behaved		
Successful or had performed well		
Ill or had hurt yourself		
Worried or anxious		
Noisy		
Worried or upset about difficulties at home		
Any others?		

Figure 3.5 Childhood connections between situations and eating

much food at home or not been able to have treats because of financial pressures. For others, it may be that they had a very strict upbringing where treats were not allowed. Whatever the reason, the sense of deprivation that can develop can lead to treats/food becoming a forbidden treasure. It changes the meaning of food.

As you can hopefully see by now, these early learning experiences and connections can become so entrenched that we aren't fully aware of them even though they drive and guide our behaviour. Our brain tries to minimise the amount of effort we put into our behaviour by taking a short cut – we subconsciously recognise a situation (e.g. upset) and then the response we have learned (eating) happens quickly and automatically. People are often deeply ashamed of this type of emotional eating after the event, but this happens when our brains have caught up and we have the benefit of hindsight. This heightened hindsight thinking is the exact opposite of automatic thinking. This is the difference between your emotional brain and your thinking brain.

Over time, as a result of this close connection between eating in response to specific emotions, we become more and more used to behaving in this way. This pattern of behaviour becomes like a well-trodden path. If we keep repeating this pattern of behaviour then it becomes our main

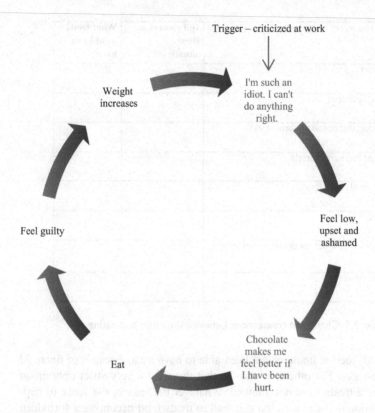

Figure 3.6 Mood and food connection

(or our only) way of coping with emotions, and so we don't get to find out that we could cope with those feelings without food. We can become deskilled or lose our skills in finding other ways of responding or coping. Our pattern of eating to manage how we feel is a smokescreen that clouds the actual issue as we give it false credit for taking away our emotional pain. We don't get to find out that we have other skills or resilience to manage these feelings regardless of whether or not we eat.

Managing your emotional eating

Introducing a pause to allow your brain to catch up

Unfortunately, we often can't control or prevent stressful life events, but we can learn how to manage and influence our own reactions to

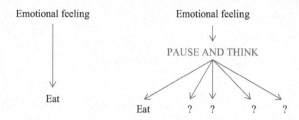

Figure 3.7 The power of the pause

these so they have less of an impact on us. To counteract our automatic responses to emotions, we need to build in a pause to allow our brains enough time to catch up, so that we can make an active choice and decision about whether eating is the most helpful thing to do in this situation. If, after pausing and thinking about it, you decide to continue, then at least you have thought it through and will hopefully feel less guilty or regretful afterwards.

To build in a pause, you have to use the information and data you have gathered earlier in this chapter about the type of emotional connections you have made with eating (e.g. eating X makes me feel Y) and identifying the typical triggers that lead to emotional eating. This will help you to recognise these situations so that you can spot yourself heading towards them.

The pause is a bit like traffic lights at a fork in the road – this is where you take a moment to stop, think and make a decision. It's a choice point. Recognise the trigger, slow down, stop and make a decision about the best way to proceed. There is the old familiar route that you can take, or you can take the alternative route which is likely to lead to a different result.

This process can help you to start regaining a sense of control and feeling that you can influence your eating.

Choosing a strategy after pausing

We are now going to start focusing on some of the other strategies that can be used to manage emotions so that you have a range of options to choose from.

It is important to include food as a possible strategy rather than deciding it is no longer an option for you. Retaining eating as one of the possible options means that people feel they have a choice to choose something

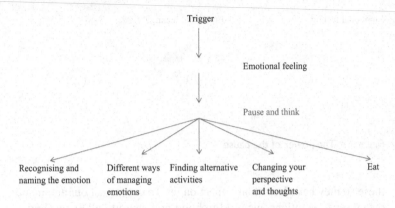

Figure 3.8 Increasing the range of strategies to manage your emotions

else. There is a risk that if you decide that eating is a "forbidden" strategy then it has the opposite effect! The aim is to develop active decision-making and to develop a range of strategies that you can choose from. If you do choose to eat, then at least you will have made an informed, considered decision rather than it being an automatic behaviour.

Recognising and naming the emotion

We often have shorthand ways of describing how we are feeling rather than naming specific emotions and making clear links between events and our emotional responses. Finding a language to identify how you are feeling and articulating the reasons for this can be a very powerful tool.

Sometimes people mislabel their physical feelings and emotional feelings. For example, a man who was pre op used to eat large amounts due to what he initially thought was hunger. However, it became clear that he was confusing anxiety and hunger. When he became anxious, he would get physical fluttery feelings in his stomach that he misinterpreted as signs of hunger and would therefore eat to manage these feelings. Just recognising and correctly labelling these physical sensations as anxiety meant that he could start to respond differently.

Strategies

Learn to label and articulate the connections behind emotional reactions – make a narrative to explain what you are feeling and what created that feeling. For example, I am feeling X because of Y. "I am feeling anxious because my boss has given me a new project to work on, and I think I will let her down."

Question the utility of food – if you take a long hard look at it, then how does food actually help with the underlying emotion or problem? What does it have to do with the underlying problem or trigger? Does the problem disappear after you have eaten?

Update your beliefs about what food does for you and disentangle past connections. Does your eating behaviour make sense in the here and now? Does it help you in the way that it might have done earlier in life?

Developing confidence in your ability to manage emotions

As discussed earlier, emotional eating responses can happen very quickly and automatically. The intensity of the emotion and threshold for responding to these emotions tends to become lower and lower over time. If you imagine rating the intensity of the emotions that affect your eating on a scale of 1 to 10, you might have initially experienced an 8/10 feeling of stress to trigger your eating. However, over time and repeated episodes of eating, this threshold reduces, so it will take lower levels of stress to trigger the eating response. This is because our brains become hyper-alert to those emotions and feelings and will notice and respond to those feelings at an earlier and earlier stage – your brain is trying to be helpful, but it's inadvertently creating a problem! It's as though your brain's early warning system has been triggered and this activates the well-established connections and beliefs that eating is a helpful way of managing that emotion.

Another problem with eating in response to emotions is that people attribute feeling better or emotions passing to eating rather than finding out that the emotions would change anyway. This strengthens the belief that eating is a helpful way of managing emotions, and this starts to guide our future behaviour (as shown in Figure 3.9).

What would happen to those feelings if you didn't eat in response to them? Emotions come and go over time – they will automatically change and pass over time, just like clouds passing in the sky. No emotion stays at the same intensity permanently. Sometimes our emotions can feel overwhelming, so eating can be a way of avoiding that feeling. People sometimes worry that if they don't eat, those feelings would become more intense and overwhelming, and this would be unbearable for them. The problem with this belief is that it keeps alive the idea that a) emotions are uncontrollable and b) eating is a way of reducing or avoiding those feelings.

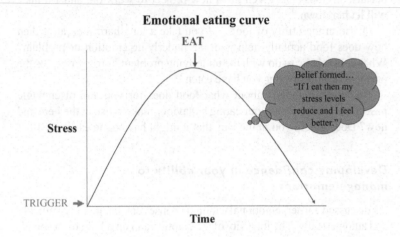

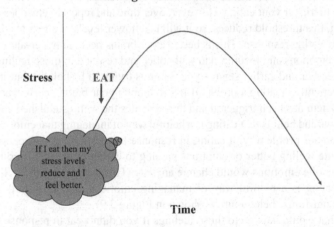

Figure 3.9 Emotional eating curve with decreasing threshold

It is important to find out what happens if you don't respond by eating when you are feeling those emotions – it's an important way to build your confidence that emotions will decrease over time and that you can tolerate emotions. If that feels too challenging, you could consider increasing the amount of time before you eat, for example, by building in a five-minute delay and then building to longer periods of time: this is building up your emotional stamina. It also allows you to find out what happens to a) the emotions that you are feeling and b) the urge to eat if you delay responding.

It can help to think of surfing the emotion – the emotion will come and go and you can just ride it out. Usually people find that when they stop avoiding or running from their emotions and allow themselves to experience them, they are much more manageable than they anticipated.

Mindfulness can also be a helpful way of building in a pause and slowing down. It can also help you to find out what happens to emotions and thoughts over time if you simply notice and observe them without getting caught up in them. There are specific mindfulness programmes and exercises available that will help you to practice and develop these skills.

Addressing and fulfilling the emotional need

When we have an emotional response, it's a signal or cue to notice what is happening – the emotion is a reflection of how we are feeling and is trying to communicate something with us. Each emotion has a specific underlying meaning or signal attached to it.

For example:

Emotion	Meaning of that emotion
Boredom	Brain needs stimulation
Loneliness	Wanting company and connection with others
Stress	Feeling overloaded by demands and unable to cope
Anger	Signals injustice and prompts you to redress this

If you attend to the underlying meaning of the emotion, it is difficult to see how food directly relates to these other than providing a distraction or avoidance. Eating does not actually address the need or resolve the problem in any way. The wrong strategy is being used in an attempt to resolve the problem. It is like someone experiencing pain when walking and deciding to use crutches when they actually need a different pair of shoes.

Once you've worked out the meaning behind the emotion and the signal it is sending you, then you can start to think about other ways of fulfilling that emotional need. This means that you are targeting your efforts at managing the emotions and the problems driving them. It also means that you avoid adding to your problems by eating and then becoming distressed about your eating and weight.

Doing the opposite of the emotion

Certain emotions tend to make us behave in certain ways – for example, if someone is feeling low or depressed then they often tend to shut down, stop doing things and hide away. Anxiety often makes people want to avoid situations so they don't have to face what worries or frightens them. The problem is that if we simply behave in accordance with our emotions, then we just reinforce how powerful they are, and we don't find effective ways of managing them. One option to consider is simply doing the opposite of what the emotion is telling you to do – so, for example, with depression you would counteract this feeling by maintaining social contact with people, going out and so on. With anxiety, you would face the situation rather than avoid it. This may sound like very simplistic advice, but it is actually a very powerful tool. It will help you to feel in control of managing your reactions to your emotions rather than the emotions simply controlling you.

Finding other things to do

Part of managing emotional eating patterns involves finding other things to do to manage your emotions. Often, people find that when they find something else to focus on or to do, the urge to eat and the emotion often subsides by itself. As mentioned previously, people have often become dependent on food as their main way of responding to these emotions, but there are all sorts of other options. These include:

- Phoning a friend
- Reading a book or magazine
- Playing computer games
- Going for a walk
- Handicrafts, e.g. knitting, making cards
- Tidying a cupboard

- Listening to music
- Doing your nails
- Doing a puzzle
- Writing a letter or email
- Having a long bath.

Build up a list of a few different things you can do when you feel the urge to eat – think of this as preparing your emergency first aid emotion kit! First try doing three of the alternative things you have identified, and if you still feel that you want to eat something after trying these, then go ahead. Most people find that the urge has passed because they have focused on something else or that their brain has had time to catch up, and they no longer feel that eating is a helpful option.

Managing thoughts that affect your emotional reactions and eating

There are two different ways in which the way we think about things can affect emotional eating patterns. We experience a trigger that we perceive or think about in a certain way and this affects our emotional reactions and feelings. Also, certain emotions affect our eating because of our past mood/food connections and the thoughts and beliefs that have developed as a result which drive us to eat.

Our thoughts are a reflection of the personal meaning and interpretation that we attach to situations. They are our own unique lens through which we view the world. Our thoughts are a reflection of our internal voice, which gives a running commentary on ourselves, others and the world, as well as making judgements and decisions. They are powerful! The way that we think about things directly affects our emotions and the way we behave. There are many different ways of viewing the same situation and your interpretation will influence how you feel and how you behave. The problem is that we tend to get stuck in certain patterns of thinking, and this affects the way we respond to situations.

The thoughts that we have sometimes whirr away at the back of our minds, and we tend not to pay much notice to them – we tend to focus on how we *feel* rather than how we think. However, if we start to identify and question how and what we are thinking then we can start to change our emotional reactions to situations. If we change our emotional reactions then we may no longer need to eat in response to these feelings.

It is helpful to identify how your thoughts affect your emotions and your eating. Shine a spotlight on your thoughts and turn the volume up on them to help you identify them and then work out if they are helpful or not. It is also helpful to evaluate whether these thoughts are an accurate appraisal of the situation.

As mentioned before, there are different levels of thoughts to target – thoughts about the trigger situation and thoughts about eating.

Thoughts about the trigger situation

Would other people see the situation in the same way?

What would you say to someone else in the same situation?

What would be a more balanced view of the situation?

Thoughts about eating

Is the belief that food helps in this situation a legacy from the past, or is it accurate?

How does food actually help the situation? How does that actually work?

How do you feel after eating? How does it make you feel about yourself? Is it worth it?

Once you can start to identify and catch these thoughts then you are in a really powerful position to start breaking out of the emotional eating cycle.

A final word . . . regular, planned eating reduces the likelihood of emotional eating

Making sure you are eating regularly is one of the most important and helpful things you can do if you are prone to emotional eating. Regular eating is as much about mood management as it is weight management. If you have big gaps in between meals then there are biological mechanisms which mean that you are highly likely to become irritable and anxious. If these happen to be your emotional triggers for emotional eating then it becomes a self-fulfilling prophecy. For some people, just starting to implement regular eating can lead to a large reduction in their emotional eating. This is an obvious place to start. At least try it so that you can only have to focus on any emotional eating patterns that are left over after addressing this.

Summary

Emotional eating is a very common problem, yet it can be very distressing and can cause problems with poor weight loss or weight regain after surgery. Trying to develop an understanding of when and where these emotional eating patterns developed and what purpose this eating behaviour has served is an important step. As a result of understanding this pattern of behaviour, it creates space for change and the possibility of responding differently in future.

References

Scholtz, S., et al. 2007. Long-term outcomes following laparoscopic adjustable gastric banding: postoperative psychological sequelae predict outcome at 5-year. *Obesity Surgery*, 17, 1220–1225.
White, M.A., et al. (2010). Loss of control over eating predicts outcomes in bariatric surgery: a prospective 24-month follow up study. *Journal of Clinical Psychiatry*, *71* (2), 175–184.

Chapter 4

Final steps before surgery

This chapter focuses on helping you to make sure that you have put things in place before surgery to make the recovery and rehabilitation period as smooth as possible. As the operation date draws closer, people often experience a mixture of excitement, apprehension and anxiety – this is completely normal and understandable. There is a blend of practical things that you need to make sure you have in place, as well as some psychological processes and issues that are likely to arise. This chapter helps you to make the final changes required before surgery and to start planning ahead for immediate changes following the operation. The aim is to put things in place now to make this as smooth a transition process as possible.

Preparing for a change in your eating

As part of their preparation for bariatric surgery, some people start to anticipate the future loss of food and the difference this may make to their life in both a positive and negative way.

It can be a process of anticipatory mourning, especially for those people whose eating has played a very important role in their life. This can often be the case for those people who are emotional eaters or where eating is a very significant part of socialising. As part of this anticipatory mourning, some will allow themselves to have certain foods that they particularly enjoy as part of a "goodbye" process. It marks the end of one type of relationship with food before another begins. For some people, it can also feel like a brief respite from dieting or weight management before having to fully commit to lifelong changes after surgery. Often people refer to this as having their "last supper" before surgery.

> Over the past few months after having an indulgent Christmas, I started getting anxiety about eating for the first time in a long time. I'm anxious about giving up all of these wonderful tastes and to be

honest, the attachment and comfort I thought I'd stopped having for them. I've had more than one ceremonial goodbye dinner. Goodbye to this, goodbye to that and I've eaten far too many sweet things. I feel a deep loss knowing "that's it, no more". I lose sleep over it. I actually mourn the pending surgery date.

LJ, 4 weeks pre op

Sometimes people can catastrophise about how life will be after surgery. They assume that they will never be able to eat socially again, that they will never be able to enjoy eating again, and that they will never be able to have occasional "treats". This is not the case. Bariatric surgery is not a punishment or condemning you to a life of purgatory. The surgery gives you a window of opportunity to redefine your relationship with food. Whilst it will involve you making major lifestyle changes, the long-term aim is for you to have a healthy, balanced relationship with food where you are satisfied after eating small amounts of food you enjoy.

Other people may have a negative, hateful relationship with food and actively dislike it because of how it has affected their weight and the impact it has had on their life. For these people, there can be a huge sense of relief that a radical change is on the horizon. The surgery provides an opportunity to "reset the body". The fact that they will have the help of an additional tool can be a huge relief for people who feel that they no longer have to keep struggling on by themselves and repeating such a painful cycle of weight loss and regain.

This is your opportunity to think about your future relationship with food. What do you want food to mean to you in future? How dominant do you want it to be in your life?

Am I making the right decision?

As the surgery date gets closer and the operation starts to feel more real, people sometimes start to doubt whether they are doing the right thing by having bariatric surgery. Making a decision to have bariatric surgery is often different to other surgical procedures because it is something that people elect or choose to have done. This is usually in contrast to other operations where people are told that they need an operation to fix a problem that has been causing clear symptoms.

Prior to surgery, some people can lose significant amounts of weight because of the changes to their lifestyle and eating they have made in preparation for it. It can be more complicated for these people, as they can start to doubt whether they really need the surgery. They may start to wonder if they can continue to lose weight if they just keep on with the same plan rather than having surgery.

This is also compounded by the societal myth that people should be able to lose their weight through dieting if only they had enough will-power. This leads some people to feel guilty and ashamed about deciding to have bariatric surgery. However, we know that it is incredibly difficult and rare for people to lose and maintain weight loss, and there are all sorts of biological mechanisms which mean that people are programmed to regain weight. The evidence is very clear that bariatric surgery is the most effective treatment for obesity. As mentioned earlier in the book, you will still have to make and maintain many changes to your eating behaviour and activity levels, but you are just boosting your chances of success. It is not an easy option. Your decision is based on very clear and compelling evidence.

This is a useful time point to remind yourself of your original reasons for seeking bariatric surgery, the issues that your weight has caused and the results of your dieting over the years.

- What were your original reasons for seeking bariatric surgery? Where did the idea come from?
- What issues has your weight led to? What has your weight stopped you from doing?
- What do you anticipate would happen to your weight and health if you do not have surgery?
- What has happened to your weight with previous diets? How long have you kept your weight off for?
- Is there anything that would be different if you were to try another diet? Do you anticipate that you could maintain it for the rest of your life?
- Is there anything you could try that you haven't? It is important to know you have exhausted all other possibilities. Most people I see have tried everything available and have put huge amounts of effort into losing weight – hence the need to add in a different tool to their skill mix.

If you are struggling with these thoughts then it is worth contacting your bariatric service to have a further discussion about your thoughts and doubts – they are in a unique position to help you think through the potential benefits and challenges you are likely to experience. They may also be able to put you in touch with someone who has had bariatric surgery to hear about their experiences. Talking to someone who has been through the surgery can be the most effective way of allaying concerns and discarding myths. Whilst online forums can be helpful, you also need to be careful as usually a selected group of people use them, and so you may get a biased view. Unless the person has had surgery through the same bariatric service, they are likely to have had a different experience. You can also talk to people who you are close to and trust about your concerns.

Managing anxiety about surgery

Most people feel anxious or worried about the prospect of having surgery. Usually their anxieties and worries are focused on having a general anaesthetic, potential complications that may occur during or after surgery and the pain they may experience afterwards. Usually people overestimate the risks of the surgery and the anaesthetic. Don't forget that bariatric surgery is a routine operation for your surgeon – they are likely to have done hundreds of these operations. They consider it equivalent to removing a gall bladder. Anaesthetists involved in bariatric surgery are usually specialists in this area and are therefore very familiar with anaesthetising people who are obese. The pre-operative assessment is put in place as an opportunity to highlight and address any concerns before the anaesthetic. There are lots of safety checks and risk assessments in place that you may not be aware of – for example, it is usual that each person having bariatric surgery will be discussed at the bariatric multidisciplinary team (with the surgeon and anaesthetist present), and any surgical and anaesthetic risks will be highlighted. For example, many people are not aware that they have obstructive sleep apnoea until they are assessed in a bariatric service. Sleep apnoea can cause ventilation and airway difficulties, and that is one of the reasons why people start treatment (usually CPAP – continuous pressure airway pressure) to optimise them for the operation. It is important that you discuss any anxieties with your bariatric team. Complications can arise after bariatric surgery, like any other operation, but they are generally rare.

Conversations about the future – disclosure and preparing others

You will need to make some decisions about how open you are going to be with other people about your upcoming surgery. People vary in terms of how private they are about having bariatric surgery. Some people prefer not to tell others about their operation, whereas others want others to be aware and to be involved in the process. There are advantages and disadvantages to both approaches. It is important to do whatever feels right for you and gives you the best chance of success going forward. Regardless of whether you decide to tell people about whether you have had bariatric surgery, it's likely that you will get some questions about changes in your eating habits and your weight loss, so you will need to be prepared for this.

This would also be a good time to start planning ahead with family and friends so that they know what to expect and don't inadvertently end up sabotaging your eating. They may need to be prepared for changes in family eating.

You may need to plan to change your socialising habits for a while, too, so that you do other things rather than going out for meals. This will make life a bit easier to begin with.

Creating a memory bank for future

The time prior to surgery is an ideal time to create a memory bank for the future. This might include taking photographs and measurements of yourself (e.g. waist, hips, thighs, arms). It is useful to take photographs of yourself standing in a doorframe, as this will provide a standard reference point that you can continue using for photos as you lose weight. You are likely to notice that the gaps around your silhouette get larger! Take some from the front and of your side profile.

These photos and measurements provide your baseline, and you can refer back to these after surgery to help you see the progress and changes you have made. These can be a particularly useful way of addressing the brain–body time lag after surgery – this is when people don't update their body image at the same speed as their weight loss. This means that people find it difficult to see that they have actually lost weight when they look in the mirror, even though they objectively know they have.

Bariatric surgery often represents a landmark moment in people's lives and they have hopes and expectations about how things will change and improve for them in future. By capturing your hopes and wishes for yourself, it can be a way of consolidating this in your mind and can be a useful thing to look back on in future. One way of doing this is to write a letter from your current self to your future self six months after surgery. In the letter, you may include:

- what you want to be different in your life
- what you want to be doing that you currently struggle with
- what you want your eating to be like

- what you want your relationship with food to be like
- your hopes about your future weight/size
- how you want your body to feel
- ways in which you want your confidence or self-esteem to change.

These are just examples of things you can include – the choice is ultimately up to you. Write the letter as though you are writing it to someone you support and are fond of. The letter is an important part of your memory bank for the future.

Smoking

If you smoke cigarettes then you need to give up before surgery. Bariatric services vary in the minimum length of time they want you to stop smoking, but the absolute minimum required is six weeks. You will not be able to resume smoking after surgery as this increases the risk of physical complications including poor wound healing and marginal ulcers, which can be very painful and serious. You will need to plan to give up smoking completely on a permanent basis.

Alcohol

Remember that it is better to avoid drinking alcohol after surgery, particularly if you have had a gastric bypass. Some people are apprehensive about how they will cope in social situations without drinking alcohol – this is particularly likely if your socialising has been based around drinking. Obviously, it is still important that you maintain your social life after surgery, but alcohol should not be part of this. It is useful to test out before surgery what it is like to engage in your usual social activities without drinking alcohol. This will help you to get used to it and will help those around you become accustomed to it as well.

Practicalities

Planning ahead

If you work, then you will need to make sure that you have planned to take time off after your operation. The amount of time off work needed varies between people and the type of job they do, but most people need to take at least two weeks off work. You will need time to recover from your operation, and it takes time and energy to get used to your new eating regime. The dramatic reduction in food intake can also add to fatigue. It might be useful to discuss a graded return to work and/or your usual activities because of the changes in your energy levels. It is important to review your commitments and responsibilities and to think about whether you need to ask for help and support from others. Also, you may need to postpone certain commitments for a while until you have recovered.

Pre-op liver shrinkage diet

The liver shrinkage diet is a very low carbohydrate and high-protein diet. You should have been given detailed guidance by your bariatric service about the liver shrinkage diet that you need to follow and the length of time that you need to follow this for. Typically, this diet needs to be followed for two weeks prior to surgery. Some individuals may be required to follow the liver shrinkage diet for longer than this, and your bariatric team will advise if this applies to you. Some services use a food-based liver shrinkage diet and others use a meal replacement option. If you use a liquid meal replacement version, make sure you are using products which are compatible with the bariatric service's requirements.

Most people having bariatric surgery have large livers – this is because the liver stores fat and a type of stored carbohydrate called glycogen. By reducing the amount of glycogen in your liver, it shrinks your liver and makes it easier for the surgeon to do the operation. The surgeon needs to move your liver during the operation to get access to your stomach. If the liver is heavy and large this can be challenging.

The liver shrinkage diet is not optional. It is an absolute requirement that you follow this diet, otherwise you run the risk of your procedure being cancelled or putting yourself at greater risk during the operation.

It is strongly recommended to give the liver shrinkage diet a trial run before surgery. It's very important to follow the diet correctly, and it is therefore important to identify any problems beforehand and seek help/advice. This will also help you to decide if you want to try the food-based liver shrinkage diet or a meal replacement liquid option. Most people find the first few days (usually three to four days) are the most challenging, and that it becomes much easier after that.

Planning for being in hospital

You will usually be in hospital for a couple of nights after your surgery (depending on the procedure), but the hospital will be able to give you guidance based on your specific circumstances. Many people find it challenging to be in hospital and want to get home as soon as possible. It is helpful to think about what you might need to take with you to make your hospital stay more comfortable and manageable. You might want to think about things that will help you pass the time – for example, reading books, puzzle books, music. Think about whether you prefer to be on your own or whether you want people to visit you.

On a practical level, you will also need to think about how you will get home after being discharged, and who will collect you.

Try to identify what type of support you might need at home and who is best placed to provide it. What sort of things would you like them to do? Equally importantly, what sort of things would you like them *not* to do?! Having these conversations ahead of the situation is likely to increase the chance of it going according to plan and gives you an opportunity to iron out different expectations.

Planning ahead for post-op eating

After surgery, you will need to follow a structured eating plan for the first couple of months. This is often referred to as the texture progression diet. It involves reintroducing different food textures gradually to avoid discomfort and reduce the risk of vomiting. It also allows the stomach time to recover and heal after surgery. You will start by having smooth liquids before moving on to puree foods, then soft food before finally reintroducing solid food. You can prepare in advance by making sure you have appropriate foods available for these different phases. Some people like to cook and freeze food in advance – for example, making soups for the liquid phase. You will need to make sure that you have small containers to freeze food in as your portion sizes will be much smaller.

It is very important to get enough protein in your diet after surgery. Low protein is a cause of fatigue, hair loss, anaemia, impaired wound healing and loss of muscle mass. Often, it is recommended that people use a protein powder after surgery to meet their nutritional requirements. It is worth trying some different ones before surgery as it can take time to find a flavour or type that you like.

Your bariatric service will advise you which multivitamins you will need to take. There are only a few multivitamins available that contain all the supplements you need, so make sure you get one of the recommended tablets. If you don't already take a multivitamin then it might be useful to start getting into a habit of taking one before surgery.

*Reminder of the "golden rules" for eating
after bariatric surgery*

There is a set of specific "golden rules" for eating after bariatric surgery
you will need to follow. It's useful to get into the habit of following these
before surgery as much as possible. The golden rules are:

- Take bites no bigger than the size of your thumbnail – it can help to
  use a teaspoon or children's cutlery when eating.
- Chew at least 20 times or until the food has become puree-texture
  before swallowing.
- Wait between bites and put your cutlery down (you should aim for
  one bite per minute).
- Stop eating after about 20 minutes.
- Avoid drinking and eating at the same time. Don't drink for 10 minutes
  before eating, and then wait for 30 minutes after eating. This will help
  avoid overfilling your stomach pouch and regurgitating. If you eat and
  drink at the same time then this means you will flush food through
  your stomach, which means you are less likely to feel full, and it can
  therefore trigger hunger.
- Sit down to eat – this will help you to avoid getting into a habit of
  grazing.

Summary

This is your final opportunity to make sure that you have everything you
need in preparation for surgery. It is worth putting the effort in now to
make these final preparations and plan ahead, as it will mean that you
have a smoother and easier recovery.

Part II

Life after bariatric surgery

The second part of the book focuses on life after bariatric surgery, both the immediate challenges and those which occur after the "honeymoon period" of automatic and rapid weight loss.

Chapter 5

Life on the other side

Adjusting to early life changes after bariatric surgery

In this chapter, we will focus on both the immediate and short-term changes and challenges that people often experience following their bariatric operation.

Getting on the road to recovery following your operation

People often find their pain and recovery isn't as challenging as they anticipated after their bariatric operation, although this does vary between individuals. Post-operative recovery time following bariatric surgery depends on many factors including the type and number of other health issues you have, your general fitness and how straightforward the operation was. The amount of support you have around the home from family and friends afterwards can also affect your recovery. For some people, their recovery can take longer than they anticipated, and this can be difficult to cope with. Sometimes this happens because they have expectations that they "should" have recovered by a particular time point and make comparisons with other people or previous operations they have had. As bariatric surgery is usually a laparoscopic keyhole operation, people often wrongly conclude that the operation is minor because the scars they have are so small. This is not the case. Weight loss surgery is a major procedure from which it can take some time for your body to fully heal. Often, people experience fatigue after surgery as a side effect of the procedure itself, as well the impact of your new eating plan, which is a shock to the system as it involves eating much smaller amounts of food than your body was previously used to.

Some tips on coping with recovery:

- **Remember, you will not always feel like this.** Recovery happens in small steps over time, and it's important to keep track and pay attention to these as sometimes they can go unnoticed. For example, what can you do this week that you were unable to do last week?
- **Everybody's pain threshold is different.** Your pain threshold is not a reflection of whether you are "soft" or "tough". If you are struggling with pain, talk to your team and they will be able to advise you about pain medication. Don't forget that you are not able to take non-steroidal anti-inflammatory pain medication after a bypass – these include ibuprofen, naproxen and diclofenac. The reason why you can't take these medications is that they increase the risk of you getting an ulcer. If you get anxious and upset about your pain and then start to focus on it, the pain is likely to get worse. This is because when people are anxious, they start to experience physical tension in their bodies (think about what happens to your neck and shoulder muscles when you are stressed), and this makes pain worse. Try to reduce the physical tension by using relaxation and breathing exercises that focus on slow, long, deep breathing.

When you are anxious or tense then your breathing is likely to speed up – it's an evolutionary mechanism for preparing to deal with danger. Relaxed breathing sends a signal to the body that it is safe to relax and helps relieve physical tension. Relaxed breathing is slower and deeper than usual breathing. The breath goes deeper towards the belly rather than just in the chest.

To practice, make sure you are sitting or lying comfortably.

- Breathe in for a count of 4. Imagine your belly as a balloon that you are gently trying to inflate – you might want to rest a hand gently on your stomach so that you can feel your stomach moving gently.
- Pause for 1.
- Breathe out for a count of 4.
- Pause for 1.
- Then repeat – 4/1/4/1.

Make sure your breathing is long, steady and continuous. Don't take a sudden intake of breath or try to hold your breath. You may discover that breathing in and out to the count of 4 is too long or short for you, so you can adapt the number to whatever helps you do slow, continuous breathing.

Figure 5.1 Breathing exercises

- **Pace yourself.** It is often helpful to gradually introduce aspects of your usual routine in order for you to start to regain a sense of normality. It is important to get the balance between encouraging your recovery and not pushing yourself too much. It is better not to make comparisons between what you can currently do and what you could previously do, as this can be demoralising. It is better to use your current functioning as your baseline and build up gradually. For example, this might involve building up from having a shower, going for a five-minute walk and then 10 minutes of household chores. The goal is to find a level of activity that you can consistently maintain on a frequent basis rather than pushing yourself one day and then needing to recover for the next couple of days before repeating the cycle.
- **Ask for/receive help from others.** Many people seeking bariatric surgery often provide care and support for other people yet find it difficult to request or accept help from others. This is the time to let others know how they can help and support you – often people are pleased to be asked! Although it is obviously preferable if people offer to help, you can't always rely on them offering to do this, so you may have to ask for help and let them know how they can help you. We tend to get stuck in roles in our relationships with one person being the provider of help and the other being the recipient of help. If you are usually the provider of help then this means that others may not be used to thinking about what they need to do to help you. It doesn't mean that they don't care or don't want to help – it's just that they aren't used to it.

Managing your energy

You are likely to notice that you are more fatigued than usual after surgery. This is because of the process of recovery, and also because your body is getting used to functioning on less food. It takes a while to reach an energy equilibrium. As mentioned previously, it is important to pace yourself so that you gradually build up your energy and stamina again.

Managing dips in mood post op

In the early stages following surgery, people may experience a dip in mood or might feel particularly emotional. This can take people by surprise as they often assume that they will feel much happier after their surgery because they have finally had their operation. There are a few different reasons for low mood following surgery. Having a general anaesthetic can affect your mood for a few weeks afterwards. Also, once someone has got over the euphoria of getting through the operation, their mood can sometimes dip when they face the reality of the work ahead. Pain can also have an impact, and it can take its toll on how we feel emotionally, especially if it means it is difficult to engage in our usual activities. If someone has a history of depression then it's also important to realise that this could be a more vulnerable time for you, so it's important to proactively plan around this, for example, seeking support from others, planning activities and so on. People may miss food they previously enjoyed during the first few weeks when they are following the texture progression diet. It is important to let people know how you are feeling so they can help you. You may want to talk to family, friends, your GP or your bariatric team.

One of the main triggers for someone's mood dipping after surgery is if they feel that their expectations have not been met and/or they are not progressing in the way they anticipated. An example of this would be if someone feels they are struggling with the post-operative diet and that they are not progressing as anticipated. For example, they may experience pain when eating or frequent regurgitation. These early bumps in the road can be difficult for people to manage. Remember that everyone's experience of recovery following bariatric surgery is individual – both in the speed that they recover from the actual operation and then in the way they cope with the post-operative eating plan.

One of the effects of low mood and depression is to make everything seem effortful, and it can be very difficult to motivate yourself to do things. This means that you may have stopped doing things that previously kept your mood lifted. This can make the recovery process much slower. This can create a vicious cycle as shown in Figure 5.2.

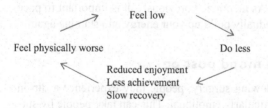

Figure 5.2 The vicious cycle of low mood and slower recovery

There is a treatment called behavioural activation, which is an important and effective way of breaking out of this vicious cycle, and evidence shows that it can really help to improve mood. Behavioural activation focuses on helping you to rebuild and increase your activity levels. Depression can also affect our ability to plan, so that can be another reason why we stop doing things. By activity, I am not referring to exercise necessarily – rather, things that we do as part of our normal daily lives. Feeling a sense of achievement and starting to re-engage with things that you enjoy are really important ways of lifting low mood. It is important to start planning small things to do every day. Not only will this help with depression, but it will also help with your physical recovery as well as regaining a sense of confidence in your body.

The way that we view and think about things is also affected by our mood. When we are feeling low, we tend to view ourselves and the world in a negative way, or we may jump to negative conclusions. Low mood leads to negative thought patterns, and these negative thought patterns then keep our mood low – yet another vicious cycle!

The thoughts that go through our minds directly influence the way we feel – they reflect our interpretation of our world, what has happened to us and what is likely to happen to us; they reflect our internal voice. The problem is that we can get stuck in a rut with these depressing thoughts, and we tend to lose perspective. If you have particular worries or thoughts that are going through your mind when you are feeling low, write them down. This can help in two ways:

1) It can help get the thoughts out of your head rather than being trapped, going round and round.
2) It can help you step back from these thoughts and influence or change your perspective.

Low mood

Negative thoughts

Figure 5.3 Low mood and negative thoughts perpetuate each other

You might find it useful to talk to family or friends about how you are feeling, as they may be able to help you see things differently. More information about how to manage low mood and negative thinking patterns can be found in Chapter 8.

Managing eating changes

It is helpful to think of the first few months after your operation as being a trial-and-error learning period as there are a number of new things to learn. These include:

- discovering how much food you can manage in your smaller stomach and adjusting your portion sizes
- adjusting your eating to follow the golden rules, e.g. eating slowly

> A few times I've found that I don't know when the last mouthful is so I've found I have to eat really slowly so that I can *feel* it more.
> VS, 4 years post surgery
> (bypass and revisional)

- identifying the foods that you are able, and unable, to tolerate (this varies between people)
- learning how to organise and manage your new eating and drinking regime into your life
- adjusting your shopping and cooking.

This stage is about discovering and educating yourself about your new digestive system and getting used to a smaller stomach. This is a work in progress, and it will take time to identify what works best for you. Whilst each person will have their own unique experience, it is important to stick to the new pattern of eating. This includes sticking to the golden rules and being mindful of your portion sizes and eating choices in order to achieve long-term weight loss. These behaviours and guidelines will help you protect your operation and get the most out of your investment. If you are struggling with any aspect of this then the dietitians in the bariatric service will be able to offer you some guidance.

Texture progression following surgery

After your operation, you will need to follow a structured eating plan. You will have to follow this plan for the first few weeks after your operation – this typically involves moving from liquids to puree foods to soft foods and then to normal texture foods. Your bariatric service will provide you with detailed information about this. It is important to stick to this plan because if you move too quickly onto the next stage, you are likely to experience pain and regurgitation. Other more serious consequences include stretching the stomach pouch and perforation. Remember, these are temporary but necessary stages to work through – stick with each stage for the appropriate time period, even though you may feel tempted to fast forward to the next stage.

Sometimes people struggle with pain and/or regurgitation when moving onto a different texture. Whilst you will have been given some guidelines about when to move onto soft foods or solid texture food, some people need to remain at certain stages for longer. If you try to move onto a new stage and find that you are not able to tolerate a particular food, think about your eating style:

Did you eat slowly?

Did you eat small mouthfuls?

Did you chew enough?

Did you sit down to eat?

It would be helpful to start keeping a diary of what it is you are eating that triggers these problems. If you continue to struggle then you should talk to your bariatric team about this, as they will be able to advise you about what steps you can take to progress. Many people find it helps to go back a stage in their texture progression (e.g. from solid texture to soft food) before trying to move forward again. Don't be put off if you find that eating something from a different texture group doesn't work the first time – try again in a while.

Sometimes people get anxious before eating, particularly if they have had a few experiences of vomiting after eating – it can become a self-fulfilling prophecy. It is easy to slip into the pattern of predicting that you will vomit, therefore tensing up, which means that it is going to be much more difficult for food to get down, hence increasing the chance of vomiting. Learning and practising some breathing exercises to help you relax can help food go down more easily as it reduces the physical tension. You can use the same breathing exercises described earlier in this chapter.

You will need to really slow down and take your time when eating. Sometimes when people are stressed about eating they eat quickly to "get it over with", and this inadvertently means they are more likely to trigger regurgitation and struggle to keep food down.

It's likely that there will always be certain foods that you struggle with after surgery – the specific type of foods varies between people, but it is important to make sure that you aren't struggling because of how you are eating or because there are any underlying physical complications with your surgery. Talk to your team about this, as they will be able to give you advice about your eating style/skills and will decide if you need any investigations.

Managing fluids

Managing your fluid intake after surgery is very important, as dehydration is the most common reason for readmission following surgery. Symptoms of dehydration include not passing much urine, dizziness or light-headedness, dry lips and skin, headaches and so on.

You should aim to have at least 1.5 litres, preferably 2 litres of low-calorie fluid per day. It can be challenging to get into a routine of eating and drinking separately at the same time as getting enough fluid in. Remember that you should not drink for 10 minutes before eating, and then you need to wait 30 minutes after eating before you have a drink. Most people need to actively work at this to ensure that they are having enough liquids.

Strategies include:
- putting time markers on your water bottle, e.g. by 11am you need to have consumed up to a certain line on the bottle
- planning how many glasses or bottles per day you need to consume
- thinking about what temperature works best for you (room temperature or warm are often easier than cold)
- considering adding flavour by adding a squeeze of lemon or no-added-sugar squash
- downloading a bariatric hydration app that will keep track of how much fluid you have consumed and remind you when to drink.

Reminder of the golden rules

After bariatric surgery, your stomach is much smaller (the size of a walnut if you've had a bypass), which means that if you continue to drink and eat as before surgery, then you will get pain and regurgitate. That is why it is important to follow the golden rules for eating after bariatric surgery.

What are the golden rules?

- Take bites no bigger than the size of your thumbnail – it can help to use a teaspoon or children's cutlery when eating.
- Chew at least 20 times or until a puree before swallowing.
- Wait between bites and put your cutlery down (you should aim for one bite per minute).
- Stop eating after about 20 minutes.
- Avoid drinking and eating at the same time. Don't drink for 10 minutes before eating and then wait for 30 minutes after eating. This will help avoid overfilling your stomach pouch and regurgitating. If you eat and drink at the same time then this means you will flush food through your stomach, which means you are less likely to feel full, and it can therefore trigger hunger.
- Sit down to eat – this will help you to avoid getting into a habit of grazing.

Prioritising the right foods

In the very early stages after bariatric surgery, hydration is the most important thing to focus on, closely followed by making sure that you are having enough protein. Most of your diet should be protein based at this point because it is needed to protect your health. Protein malnutrition can lead to physical symptoms such as hair loss, skin issues, lethargy and fatigue. If you are eating a high-protein diet whilst you are losing weight then it allows you to lose fat rather than muscle, which means that in the long term, you are more likely to maintain your health. Your body composition should retain a good proportion of muscle in order to keep your metabolism working effectively.

You may want to use protein shakes to begin with as this can help with hydration and getting enough protein in. When eating a meal, make sure you prioritise the protein on the plate. If you imagine dividing your small plate into the different food groups then you should aim for half your portion to be protein. Focus on the protein, followed by salad or vegetables and finally, carbohydrates.

Managing portion sizes

The dietitian in the bariatric service will be able to give you feedback on your portion sizes. Following a bypass, your stomach is the size of a walnut, so you will only be able to manage a few mouthfuls of food at first (around the equivalent of a few tablespoons of food). Over time, you will be able to eat a little more, but your meal size will still be much smaller than before surgery. Usually people's portion sizes increase to the point where they eat from a tea plate or side plate – this will become your new normal portion size. If you eat larger portions then it is possible to stretch the stomach pouch over time and this can lead to weight regain.

Getting into a routine and eating regularly

It helps to take a "project management" approach to planning your eating and drinking – there are many requirements to meet, and so you need to spend time working out how you can factor them all in. It can be quite a challenge to fit them around a busy lifestyle!

Bariatric surgery affects the gut hormones (ghrelin and leptin) that make us feel hungry and full. This means that after surgery, some people don't experience hunger, and so you may not experience a physical cue to eat. In fact, some people describe going all day without eating without really noticing this. This can lead to skipping meals and not eating enough of the right foods to maintain your health. This lack of hunger and desire to eat can feel like a very strange and novel experience. For some people it can be a relief that they no longer have to manage their thoughts about food or hunger any more, but it can lead to problems with not eating enough. Many people have been on diets previously where they have been told "don't eat unless you are hungry", so it can feel very strange and wrong to then have to push yourself to eat when you don't feel hungry. It is important to get into an eating routine because you may not get internal cues of hunger that trigger you to eat. This is about proactively managing your eating to make sure you are getting the right foods at the right time.

- You could consider setting yourself regular times to eat (rather than relying on your stomach to remind you).
- Set alarms on your phone as a prompt.
- Ask others to remind you to eat.
- Carry foods and snacks with you.

There are various issues and complications associated with skipping meals and eating irregularly. If you have large gaps between eating then you are likely to experience low blood sugar, which causes headaches, fatigue and difficulties concentrating. Eating irregularly is also likely to contribute to problems with constipation (a common problem for many people in the early period following surgery). Skipping meals also puts you at greater risk of nutritional deficiencies and not getting enough nutrition to maintain your health. Most people seek bariatric surgery because they want to improve their health and quality of life – eating regularly is an important part of this.

Changes in shopping and cooking

There are some practical changes to be made with your food shopping and cooking after bariatric surgery.

Obviously, you may have to change the type of foods that you shop for, particularly to make sure that you are getting enough protein-rich foods.

Think about the type of foods you tend to have around you – what foods do you store at home? If you need to grab something in a hurry, what sort of foods would you have available? You will also need to think about having snacks that you can carry around to help with regular eating and help you avoid making inappropriate food choices. Psychologist Kelly Brownell suggests we should focus on planning our food shopping and environment in order to set "optimal defaults". This means we make sure that we have the right foods easily available.

The amount of food that you will need to purchase will decrease, and it can take a while to get used to buying the right amount. People often end up buying too much food at first and end up wasting it. This can be difficult for some people to tolerate (especially those who grew up being told it was "wrong to waste food"), so they end up overeating. To ensure you are eating portions that are appropriately sized after surgery, you may find it helpful to divide meals into small portions and freeze them for later. Most people find that it's better to avoid making large amounts of food as this can set up an overeating or grazing pattern if it is easily available. If you do cook more than you need then package it up as soon as possible and use it for lunch the next day or freeze it.

There are different challenges for those who live alone versus those who live as part of a family. For those that live alone, getting used to preparing and cooking such small portions and buying the right amount of food required can take time. If you are used to preparing and cooking

food as part of a family then this can also create some issues. It is important to talk to your family about your new eating plan and whether they
are going to follow the same pattern or eat differently.

Initial weight loss

The initial weight loss after your surgery can be very rapid and dramatic.
This can be very exciting as it's what people have wanted for a long
time, but it can also be quite shocking at the same time. This is how one
woman described her reaction to her weight loss in the first couple of
weeks after her operation:

> The weight was coming off so quickly . . . my clothes were getting
> too big for me in just a two-week period, it was just coming off
> so fast . . . I was just astounded every time I got weighed. It was
> exciting but shocking as well. Initially the surgeon said it would be
> 12 months of losing weight and I thought 'oh my god, I'm going to
> end up really thin' . . . and then I thought because I'm losing it so
> quickly does that mean that in a few months I'm going to put it all
> back on again?
>
> GC, 4 months post bypass

This initial period of rapid weight loss can be exhilarating and feels
almost magical for some people. It can be compelling for people to keep
weighing themselves every day, as there are often losses every day,
initially. This experience of rapid daily/weekly weight loss is such a
powerful, almost addictive experience for people who have struggled
with their weight. Obviously, you can't continue to lose weight at the
same rate, and there will be a time when weight loss slows or you reach a
plateau for a while, so it's important to be prepared for this. Weight loss
happens in steps, not a straight line.

The way in which you react to your weight loss slowing or temporarily
stopping is important – it can have an impact on your mood and eating.
For example, some people get very anxious and blame either themselves
("I've messed it up!") or the operation ("It's not going to work!"), which
leads to them abandoning the eating plan. Or, they panic and go back into
a dieting mindset of restriction/deprivation, which then has the opposite
effect of leading to uncontrollable cravings. It is completely natural and
normal for weight loss to slow and/or plateau – your body needs time to
catch up after a period of rapid weight loss. Your body is protecting itself
by putting the brakes on until it feels it is safe to continue losing again.

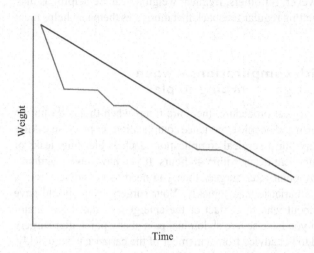

Figure 5.4 Weight loss happens in steps rather than a straight line

Obviously, when your weight loss slows or stops you should still monitor and review your eating patterns and behaviour to make sure that you are on track and following the rules. If you are on track and your weight has slowed/got stuck then just continue what you have been doing; your body will catch up and you will start to lose again. If you find you have gone off track, this is your prompt to refocus on the bariatric eating plan.

Try to avoid making comparisons with others about how much weight they have lost over certain time periods. These comparisons can lead to people feeling anxious that they aren't losing weight quickly enough or that they are doing something "wrong". Different people will have different rates of weight loss after surgery. Furthermore, your pre-surgery weight will affect how much weight you lose; that is, those who are heavier tend to lose more weight initially. Be careful of social media sites – whilst they can be a useful source of support, they can often lead to people making unhelpful comparisons with others about the amount of weight that they have lost over a specific time period (or with a particular type of surgery).

It can be tempting for people to weigh themselves every day, especially when they are going through the phase of rapid weight loss. You need to work out the frequency that works best for you. If you weigh yourself too frequently then you are likely to pick up small fluctuations in your weight (both up and down) that could be distracting or send you off track. However, for others, frequent weighing can be helpful as they feel they are getting regular feedback that motivates them and helps them stay on track.

Coping with complications – when things don't go according to plan

As with any surgical procedure, there are times when things do not go according to plan and people experience complications or problems. After bariatric surgery, most surgical complications such as bleeding, leaks or pulmonary embolism occur within 48 hours. If you have severe abdominal pain at any point after surgery then you need to get advice from a member of the bariatric team quickly. Your surgery team should have advised you about who to contact or the emergency plan if any major issues arise. If you have severe abdominal pain at any point after surgery then you need to get advice from a member of the bariatric team quickly. Also, if you experience heat and swelling in your legs or shortness of breath, seek advice urgently.

If you are vomiting frequently then it is important to let your bariatric team know, as it can cause problems and you may require additional supplementation to avoid associated complications. Other difficulties include not being able to manage enough food or liquid – again, it's important to let your team know so that they can work with you to help you through this phase.

It is important to contact your bariatric team if you have any concerns/issues.

Summary

This period of recovery after bariatric surgery is an important time to establish firm foundations for your future behaviour and weight loss. The process of recovery and adjustment will vary between people. There are many different changes to adjust and adapt to simultaneously, and this may feel overwhelming. However, it will get easier over time as you work through the texture progression plan and develop a routine that works for you. It is really important to stick to the guidance that the bariatric team has provided and seek help if you are struggling.

Chapter 6

Negotiating weight changes after bariatric surgery
The honeymoon period and beyond

This chapter focuses on the different stages of weight loss that people experience after bariatric surgery. The first stage is the honeymoon period, which is characterised by rapid weight loss which then slows until there is a transition into weight maintenance. The final section focuses on dealing with setbacks and how to get back on track.

Rapid weight loss phase

Following bariatric surgery, the speed of weight loss varies between people (and depends on the type of operation), but it is usually much more rapid than with previous diets. This weight loss can create mixed emotions. It can feel exhilarating at first, but it can also feel shocking as the speed of weight loss may feel uncontrollable and unstoppable.

It felt like being on a very fast rollercoaster at times. The weight loss was both exciting but also shocking – I couldn't believe how much my weight was changing within weeks and how quickly I was going through clothes sizes. It felt very different to any time when I had lost weight before. I was excited but there were times when I was worried that I would continue to lose weight at the same rate.

GC, 4 months post bypass

Some people start to worry that because they are losing weight so quickly, this will continue and it won't stop. This can be particularly anxiety provoking and unsettling for people who like to feel in control of situations as it can feel like their weight loss is running away with them.

Obviously when the weight first started coming off it was amazing, just brilliant. There was a point where it started to feel scary when I reached the lowest weight that I'd reached on a diet before and I was going beyond it. It suddenly started to feel a bit scary. It was terrifying because I didn't know how to slow it down. I didn't know how to deal with other people's reactions to that rapid weight loss too as I was struggling to manage my own fears. I just had to trust my body and had to go with it . . . you can't control it at this point and you just have to trust that your weight will settle where it will settle.

AM, 10 months post bypass

The quotations above illustrate that in the early weeks and months after the operation, it usually feels like the surgery is driving the weight loss. Weight loss at this stage feels automatic and just seems to happen regardless of the person's behaviour – this has often been described as the honeymoon phase.

Back to reality with a bump . . . weight loss plateaus

There will be a point at which your weight loss starts to slow, and it may plateau or stop. During the early phase of weight loss, it is easy to fall into the trap of expecting that weight loss is just going to continue with daily or weekly changes. However, it is inevitable (and completely normal) that there may be no weight loss for a few weeks even though you continue to follow the same eating pattern. The body needs time to catch up with itself and recalibrate. Sometimes people panic at this point and wonder whether they have lost all the weight they will lose or think that something is wrong with the operation or that they have done something wrong – in fact, it's none of those things; it's just part of the process. Remember, as discussed in Chapter 5, weight loss following surgery happens in steps: it is not a straight downward line. You just have to stay on track and continue to do what you have been doing, and your body will catch up with you.

A very large American study (Courcoulas et al. 2013) followed the weight loss of people for three years after their bariatric surgery and found that the majority of people got to their lowest weight one year after surgery. However, they identified different patterns of weight loss which started to emerge around six months after surgery. They identified five different patterns of weight loss from this six-month point, which included some people who continued to lose weight as well as others who started to plateau or even regain weight.

Too fast or too slow? Losing weight at the right pace

Sometimes people can be in a hurry to lose their excess weight as quickly as possible, and they put a lot of pressure on themselves to do this. This means that they can end up becoming too obsessed with their eating and weight. As a result, their emotional health and quality of life suffers.

> I want to reach the target weight I have set myself as soon as possible – I can only really settle when I get there. I have invested so much in this operation I need to make sure it works. I can't allow for any slip-ups or mistakes. The week when I don't lose any weight is going to be devastating and I will just have to get stricter with myself.
>
> SP, 6 months post sleeve gastrectomy

Remember, it is not a weight loss race! There will be individual differences in the rate of weight loss – this is about losing weight at the right speed for you. It is important to pace your weight loss as this gives your body and your mind time to catch up too. Problems can also arise when people start making comparisons with other people who have had bariatric surgery. Your bariatric team will be able to give you feedback about whether you are on track or losing weight too quickly.

It is important to remain realistic about your likely weight loss over time. The clinic should be able to estimate what they think your weight range is likely to be after surgery. These estimates are based on research looking at the weight loss of thousands of people who have had bariatric surgery. However, sometimes people forget or ignore these estimates and become unrealistic with the weight loss targets they set themselves. Remember that after a gastric bypass, a successful result is likely to lead to you losing 75% of your excess weight, but this means that you will still be 25% overweight (i.e. 25% over a BMI of 25).

When thinking about weight targets that you set yourself, you can check how realistic they are by asking yourself:

- When were you last that weight? How old were you? How many people do you know who are lighter at their current age compared to when they were younger?

Don't get distracted or obsessed by the numbers on the scales. Numbers are just numbers. There is sometimes a danger that people will start shifting their weight loss targets and goals over time – once they have reached a certain weight they were aiming for, they set themselves a new goal and the process goes on! Remember that the numbers on the scales are meaningless in themselves – what truly matters is what this weight loss enables you to do in your life.

Frequency of weighing

It is helpful to weigh yourself regularly so that you get some feedback about what is happening with your weight so that you can gauge whether you are on track or need to adjust your eating behaviour or activity levels. The traditional advice is to weigh just once per week, but there is some new evidence that daily weighing is more beneficial. However, problems sometimes arise with daily weighing if people get stressed or catastrophise about the minor, normal weight fluctuations that we all experience. Most people's weight varies by 1–2kg per day (although it can be up to 4–5kg in people with specific health conditions). Any fluctuations you notice on a daily basis are likely to be related to a combination of eating, drinking, constipation, hormonal factors, activity levels and so on.

People generally focus on the amount of weight they still have to lose rather than what they have achieved so far. It is helpful to use a weight chart to look at weight changes over time so that you can put your overall weight loss into context by looking at the big picture. This helps when your weight loss stops or slows.

Sometimes I worry that I am not doing well enough because my weight loss has slowed down. I have a graph of my weight that I've kept since I first started being seen in the bariatric surgery clinic and it really helps to look back at where I started and where I've got to now. When I look at it, I can see that I have lost a huge amount of weight and it spurs me on to keep going. There might be times when I've had a little blip where my weight has gone up slightly or I've not lost weight but looking at the overall weight loss helps me to put it in perspective and stay focused on what I have to do.

TS, lost 120kg pre and post sleeve

If you plot your weight on a graph, this can help you identify the direction and speed of your weight loss over time – it's a better representation of your weight than just the numbers on the scales. The weight graph enables you to join the dots up to make a coherent picture.

Accepting stability of weight

Most people who have bariatric surgery have lost large amounts of weight previously only to regain it within a short period of time. Most people who have yo-yo dieted do not have any experience of their weight remaining stable, as they are either losing weight or regaining weight and there is usually nothing in between. Often people have lost trust in themselves and their bodies because of their previous experiences of weight loss and weight regain. It can be anxiety provoking and difficult to believe that the same cycle won't occur after surgery. This can become more of a pressing issue as people get closer to the lowest weight they have previously been as they may expect this to be the point at which their weight regain starts.

Recognising and trusting that you can remain weight stable after surgery is a novel experience. The process of losing weight after bariatric surgery is different to weight loss on a diet. Surgery works differently because it changes your anatomy and gut hormones. But also, this is because you are not on a diet after surgery (as you know, these tend to be temporary): you are making lifelong sustainable changes to your eating. This is about re-educating your body and developing trust in it.

Worrying about weight regain leading to undereating

Some people become very worried about the possibility of weight regain after bariatric surgery, and this leads to restrictive eating and an obsessive focus on their weight. People who experience this difficulty tend to lose more weight than we would expect (usually in a shorter period of time too). Some people may also deliberately make themselves vomit or use laxatives as a way of "getting rid of" calories. They may have a distorted body image, still viewing themselves as being very overweight despite the fact that they have lost more weight than would be expected. This anxiety about weight and these behaviours can start to mimic those experienced by people with eating disorders like anorexia or bulimia. Sometimes people find it difficult to accept that they may be at risk of developing an eating disorder as they assume that someone needs to be underweight to have anorexia (this is no longer the case). Sometimes people want to continue losing more weight because they believe that this additional weight loss will then create a buffer, so that if they do regain some weight, they will still be in a weight range that is acceptable to them.

I would weigh myself all the time – if my weight went up even by a tiny bit then I would stop eating because I was so terrified that my weight would just start to go up really quickly. I had to try to put the brakes on my weight. I would eat just tiny amounts every day . . . often just one small meal every day or sometimes I would just drink tea so that I didn't have to have anything to eat. I started to feel like that wasn't working and then I started making myself sick after every meal.

AG, 3 years post bypass

There is not much information about how frequently this problem occurs, but it is certainly underreported and underrecognised as a problem. One study (de Zwaan et al. 2010) found that 12% of people who have had bariatric surgery make themselves vomit as a way of trying to lose weight.

When is it time to seek help with this problem? You should seek help if you have a fear of regaining weight, which means you restrict your eating intake to below clinical recommendations in order to lose weight quicker (sometimes this may involve not eating for a day or just eating one meal per day). If you find that you are becoming obsessive about your weight and weighing yourself frequently then this is also an indication of problems. It is very important to seek help to address this problem, as it can be very distressing and dangerous.

What is the right weight for you? Who decides and how do you decide?

The terminology we use to describe weight loss after bariatric surgery can be confusing. It's important to understand this as otherwise people can misinterpret information and feel that they have not lost as much weight as they "should" have done. We calculate the percentage of excess weight loss (commonly referred to as %EWL) to describe the amount of weight lost after bariatric surgery and to be able to estimate whether someone is on track in terms of what we would expect after surgery. This term refers to the difference between your initial weight before surgery and what your weight would be if you had a BMI of 25 (the top end of the "healthy range"). If you were to get to a BMI of 25, you would have lost 100% of your EWL. However, after bariatric surgery, we do not expect that someone will lose 100% of their EWL. We expect that if someone has a good outcome they will lose around 75% of their excess weight after a bypass, 70% after a sleeve gastrectomy and 50% following insertion of a gastric band. Remember, this is the percentage of your excess weight (over BMI 25), not your total weight. It is very important to be clear about this information as otherwise people can conclude that they have not lost enough weight and feel that they have failed. Your bariatric team should be able to calculate individual weight estimates for you based on your weight and the type of surgery you are having.

Your bariatric service will be able to help you keep track of your EWL after surgery. Or if you want to work it out yourself, you can use an EWL calculator on the internet if you know your pre-surgery weight and height.

These figures give an idea about the typical weight loss you can expect after bariatric surgery and can provide a useful benchmark. However, it is important not to be overly focused on them. Ultimately, this is about working out what is the right weight for you to be able to do the things that you want to do and to live your life in the way that you wish to.

It is important to consider other factors that might affect your weight loss, as well. For example, someone who needs to use a wheelchair is not likely to lose as much weight as someone who can mobilise without much difficulty. Certain medications may also affect your weight loss. The numbers can be useful guides, but ultimately, it is more helpful to think about your underlying reasons and future goals for losing weight. For example, a woman who had below average weight loss (about 30%EWL) after having a gastric band inserted was very happy with this outcome as it was the first time in her life that she had ever been weight stable. She predicted that if she hadn't had the surgery, her weight would have continued to increase, so from her perspective, she felt that the surgery had prevented her difficulties from worsening.

Remember your reasons for wanting to lose weight: what were they? How close or far away are you to achieving those goals? Most people don't have goals that are directly related to being a particular weight; their goals usually focus on wanting to improve their health, increasing their activity levels and their confidence and so on. It is not usually about the numbers on the scales themselves, but about what the weight loss will enable you to do or what it will improve in your life.

Accepting that you have reached your weight loss nadir

For most people who have had bariatric surgery, there comes a point where they shift towards accepting that they have lost most of the weight they are going to lose. Obviously, this is easier if your expectations have been met and you have lost as much weight as you had hoped to. It can still be challenging to allow yourself to accept your weight and to focus on weight stability/maintenance rather than pushing on to lose more weight. Each person is going to have their own individual view on what is the right size and weight for them. Sometimes people have to give themselves permission to accept that they are happy with the weight they have got to, and that it isn't necessary or helpful to keep pushing on.

If you are contemplating whether you want to focus on further weight loss versus stabilising your weight, it may be helpful to work through the following questions:

- If you maintain your current weight, how would you feel?
- What compromises would you have to make to lose more? Would you be prepared to make these, and could you sustain these?
- Who are you losing weight for?
- What would be different if you lose more weight?

It is obviously more challenging to accept your new weight if you have not lost as much as you hoped, and there is more information on dealing with this in Chapter 12.

Shifting to successful weight maintenance

Most people who have bariatric surgery are yo-yo dieters and have lost and regained weight on numerous occasions. As a result of these experiences of struggling to maintain weight loss, they aren't very confident in their (or their body's) ability to remain weight stable after losing weight.

There are physical and metabolic adjustments that present weight challenges over time. There is convincing evidence that hormonal and metabolic mechanisms mean that the body tries to defend (or return) to its highest weight. As a response to weight loss, hunger tends to increase and energy expenditure reduces, which means that the body actively tries to defend (or get back to) its higher level of body fat. It is important to be aware and realistic about these mechanisms so that you know what you need to do to counteract them to maintain your weight. We tend to assume that weight maintenance will just happen naturally rather than being something that we need to be proactive about and to focus our attention on. The skills required to maintain weight are often different to those required to lose weight.

In the next section, we focus on the behaviours that have been found to be important in maintaining weight loss. If you adopt these behaviours and embed them into your daily life then you should feel confident that your weight loss will be maintained. The idea is to make these key behaviours as transparent as possible so that you have a clear benchmark against which you can assess your own behaviour.

What behaviours do people who maintain their weight loss adopt?

Most of the information that we have about the behaviours associated with weight loss maintenance comes from research in general weight management rather than bariatric surgery specifically. However, the principles still apply. The National Weight Control Registry, based in the United States, was developed to identify people who successfully maintain weight loss and the key strategies they use to help them achieve this. In their research, they followed people who had lost at least 10% of their total body weight for 10 years to look at the common behaviours of those who keep their weight off (Thomas et al. 2014). There appear to be consistent and key behaviours that are associated with success.

These behaviours are:

- high levels of physical activity
- weighing self regularly and monitoring dietary intake
- high levels of focus and restraint
- low-calorie intake
- low levels of disinhibition therefore avoiding impulsive food choices etc.

Slipping into negative behaviours (essentially these are the opposite of those listed above) over the first 12 months was associated with weight regain over the 10-year period. The good news is that their research also shows that weight loss maintenance becomes less effortful over time, so if you manage to keep the weight off in the early years then you are more likely to keep it off longer term.

Specific skills after bariatric surgery

Maintaining awareness of your eating and weight

This is one of the foundations of weight maintenance. Keeping food diaries (or some other means of monitoring your dietary intake) and tracking your weight have consistently shown to be associated with avoiding weight regain (Odom et al. 2010). You can monitor your eating and activity by keeping diaries or using an online app. Using these tools will help you to be fully aware of your eating and drinking choices and the impact these have on your weight. It sets up a cycle where you can subsequently modify your behaviour in response to feedback from the diaries or scales.

There also seems to be evidence that those people who monitor their dietary intake and weight show more restraint with their diet and stick to the plan because they are more aware of their choices and the consequences of them.

> I need to keep track so that I can make sure I am doing the right things today for the long term.
>
> ER, 15 months post bypass,
> lost 63.6kg

It is important to weigh yourself regularly and to track your weight over time. However, it is up to you to decide the frequency that you weigh yourself – as long as you do it regularly. Traditionally, we have recommended that people weigh themselves once per week on the same day, at the same time and on the same scales. However, there is more recent evidence which indicates that for some people, it may be more helpful and effective to weigh themselves more frequently (even daily). Ultimately, it's up to you to work out the frequency that works best for you and find a frequency that strikes a middle ground between being regular enough to give you helpful feedback but not so often that it becomes obsessive.

Adherence to the long-term bariatric eating plan

It may seem like an obvious thing to say, but sticking to the long-term eating plan after surgery is critical. The research clearly demonstrates that people who do not stick to the long-term eating plan tend to regain weight. Calorie intake can increase gradually over time, and this is associated with weight regain.

One study found that those people who failed to change their eating habits after surgery were twice as likely to have poor weight loss. Another study (Sarwer et al. 2008) tracked people before and after their bariatric surgery and looked at the effect of dietary adherence on weight loss after surgery. They found differences in levels of adherence to the eating plan at just 20 weeks (4–5 months) after surgery. Those people who were adherent to the eating plan 20 weeks after their bariatric operation lost more weight over the next 18 months. Those who were non-adherent consumed more calories overall and got more calories from sweets.

This research emphasises the importance of making sure you are following the plan in the short term and long term in order to avoid weight regain. Having said that, we are not aiming for 100% perfection – this is about being "good enough, most of the time". Aiming for 90%, not 100%, is more manageable and realistic. Knowing that you have a little "wiggle room" with the remaining 10% often enables people to stay on track for the remaining 90%.

How can you be sure that you are following the plan?

- Continue to access the support of your bariatric service – being seen regularly and frequently in the first few years after your operation is associated with better outcomes.
- Be honest with the bariatric team about what is going well and what you are struggling with. Sometimes people worry that these struggles mean that they are "failing" or that they are a "bad patient" – this is not the case. The team will expect to hear about struggles, so it won't be a surprise to them!
- Keep reminding yourself of the dietary guidelines – food choices, portions and the golden rules.
- Plan your eating ahead.
- Share your food diary with someone from the bariatric team and ask for feedback.
- Be careful of underestimating dietary intake – remember that much of our eating behaviour is automatic and out of our awareness.
- Be clear that at this stage in your bariatric journey, you can no longer "get away with" eating inappropriate foods and still lose weight.

Watch out for problem eating patterns

There are certain problem eating patterns to be particularly aware of following surgery because they are associated with less weight loss. These patterns are grazing and binge eating patterns. These issues deserve more attention so there is more information on how to identify and manage these behaviours in Chapter 7. The best way of avoiding slipping into these patterns is to have a structured, regular eating plan with clear gaps in between meals.

Activity

Physical activity is an important part of the toolkit for maintaining weight loss. As the body becomes accustomed to functioning on fewer calories and its lower weight, the metabolism slows down to try and get back to the previous higher weight – it is obviously not wise or realistic for people to keep restricting their food intake more and more. This means that the main way to manage an energy balance is through increasing the amount of physical activity. Chapter 9 contains detailed information about recommendations for activity and ways that you can overcome barriers to activity.

Maintain motivation by remembering your reasons for weight loss

Over time, it is easy to lose sight of the reasons why weight loss was so important and the impact of weight problems before surgery. Our memories fade quickly sometimes! It is helpful to have your reasons for wanting to lose weight and the goals that you set yourself clear in your mind, as these can continue to motivate you to work at maintaining your achievements. These are precious achievements and are hard fought for, so need to be protected!

This also means recognising weight loss maintenance as an achievement in its own right. This is a bit of a mental shift for many people as they are so used to focusing on weight loss. The obesity doctor, Holly Wyatt, points out the fact that nobody ever compliments us on maintaining and staying the same weight! We tend to only get positive feedback about weight loss. It is therefore important to acknowledge and give yourself credit for counteracting a lot of physical and metabolic obstacles which would naturally make your weight increase.

Attending regular appointments as part of your follow-up care

Maintaining regular appointments with the bariatric service is very important as it helps people stay on track. Research shows that those people who attend regular appointments after their surgery have a better outcome and have less risk of weight regain (Odom et al. 2010).

People can sometimes be tempted to avoid from the bariatric service if they are struggling, but this is the very best time to attend – the team are there to support you and will be able to help you work out a plan to get back on track. If the team know about your struggles, they are in a much better position to be able to help you, and after all, that is what they are there to do!

Importance of support

You will be aware by now that bariatric surgery presents challenges as well as opportunities, and it is important to have support along the way to help you through. If you think about the people in your network, who is best placed to support you? It is important to identify people who will continue to encourage and motivate you. They can also remind you of the progress and changes you have made over time – it can be easy for you to lose sight of these.

Aside from your network of close relationships, it may be useful to think about attending a bariatric support group. The bariatric surgery service that you attend may run one, or there may be other voluntary organisations that provide them. A few studies have found that attending bariatric support groups is associated with better weight loss (Sheets et al. 2014).

Mental health factors

It is important to work on maintaining your psychological wellbeing at the same time as maintaining your weight. This is important because the research shows us that people who experience mental health difficulties after surgery are more likely to experience poor weight loss or weight regain. These psychological difficulties can be new problems or more often, a re-emergence of previous problems. This relationship between psychological difficulties and poor weight loss/weight regain works in both directions. Disappointing weight loss (or weight regain) and unmet expectations can be very distressing and cause psychological problems. There is also some evidence that psychological problems can lead to poorer weight loss, too (Kinzl et al. 2006; Sheets et al. 2014). There is more information about how to work on your psychological wellbeing and psychological difficulties in Chapter 8. It is worth highlighting at this point that if you are having psychological or mental health difficulties, it is important to seek help from your bariatric service or speak to your GP.

Managing behavioural drift and setbacks

It is inevitable and natural that at some point you will have a lapse or setback in terms of sticking to the eating and activity plan. It is practically impossible to stick to the plan 100% of the time, and it is unhelpful to aim for this. There are many different requirements to follow after bariatric surgery, and there are times when it is more challenging to manage all of these. We all go off track at times – we are only human! It is what you do in response to going off track that matters.

We can go off track in response to a specific life event, or we can just gradually drift back into old habits and stop practising the more recent behaviours we have learned and implemented. Sometimes we are simply overloaded with other commitments and responsibilities and we therefore can't pay as much attention to the eating plan.

Strategies

Identify your early warning signs of drift

It helps if you can spot that you have gone off track earlier rather than when it has become a more entrenched pattern. This is where the self-monitoring of your eating, activity and weight can be really helpful – you will get feedback much sooner and you can then modify your behaviour. Sometimes people are tempted not to monitor themselves when they have gone off track, as though they are convincing themselves that because it's not being recorded, it's not really happening!

There may be certain behaviours that you stop doing and others that you start doing when you are starting to go off track. If you can work out which behaviours you have started doing, and those which you have stopped doing, this information can alert you to problems sooner in future. The behaviours that are associated with being "off track" tend to stay the same over different episodes as people revert to previous patterns. Once you have identified these behaviours, they can act as early warning signs that prompt you to take action at an earlier stage of being off track.

Keeping setbacks in perspective

Sometimes, when people feel that they have lapsed or gone off track, they can become highly self-critical and have feelings of failure, shame and hopelessness. It can tap into previous experiences of yo-yo dieting, which may have led to low levels of confidence in their ability to implement long-term changes. It is important to manage your reaction to being off track because sometimes these reactions can send people further off track.

I've learnt that if I mess up once, not to beat myself up too much . . . I tell myself that I just have to start again. Who is perfect in this world? As long as I keep on trying and doing the best I can, then I am happy.

CK, 4 years post band

How far off track are you in reality? What's the evidence? If you look at the evidence, are you really off track, or could it be a fearful prediction?

Your internal conversation

What sort of internal conversations are you having about being off track? Are you behaving like a sergeant major shouting and berating yourself? In my experience, the "sergeant major" approach of shouting at yourself to motivate yourself to get back on track doesn't work. It tends to paralyse people.

Are you a doom and gloom merchant? Some people tend to catastrophise about any setbacks or signs that they have gone off track. They may think to themselves, "I've blown it all . . . I'm a complete failure". This approach tends to lead to people abandoning and disengaging from the plan as they feel hopeless that anything they do will make a difference.

Finding an alternative voice

How would you speak to a friend who wanted to get back on track? How would you encourage and support them? This doesn't mean you are "letting yourself off the hook" and not holding yourself accountable – it's about treating yourself in a way which is more likely to encourage and motivate you and believe that it is possible and manageable to get back on track.

Start taking small steps to get back on track

Once you have identified the behaviours that you have stopped and started doing since being off track, the next step is to think about introducing some small changes to help you get back on track. It is better to focus on making a few small changes rather than trying to change everything all at once. This is about rebuilding your confidence in your ability to get back on track, so it's important that you start making changes in a gradual way and give yourself credit for re-engaging.

Summary

There are different speeds and phases of weight loss after bariatric surgery. It is not realistic (or wise) to expect that the rapid weight loss that often occurs in the honeymoon phase immediately after bariatric surgery will continue. It is normal for your weight loss to slow down, and it is important that you are proactive in using strategies to maintain your weight loss rather than just assuming it will naturally happen. It is also helpful to be prepared for the fact that setbacks are normal – it is how you respond to them that truly matters and determines your long-term success.

References

Courcoulas, A.P. et al., 2013. Weight change and health outcomes at 3 years after bariatric surgery among individuals with severe obesity. *JAMA*, 310 (22), 2416–2425.

Kinzl, J.F. et al., 2006. Psychosocial predictors of weight loss after bariatric surgery. *Obesity Surgery*, 16 (12), 1609–14.

Odom, J. et al., 2010. Behavioral predictors of weight regain after bariatric surgery. *Obesity Surgery*, 20 (3), 349–356.

Sarwer, D.B. et al., 2008. Preoperative eating behavior, postoperative dietary adherence, and weight loss after gastric bypass surgery. *Surgery for Obesity and Related Diseases*, 4 (5), 640–646.

Sheets, C.S. et al., 2014. Post-operative psychosocial predictors of outcome in bariatric surgery. *Obesity Surgery*, 25 (2), 330–345.

Thomas, J.G. et al., 2014. Weight-loss maintenance for 10 years in the national weight control registry. *American Journal of Preventive Medicine*, 46 (1), 17–23.

de Zwaan, M. et al., 2010. Comprehensive interview assessment of eating behavior 18–35 months after gastric bypass surgery for morbid obesity. *Surgery for Obesity and Related Diseases: Official Journal of the American Society for Bariatric Surgery*, 6 (1), 79–85.

Chapter 7

Negotiating your new relationship with food and managing pitfalls

The first part of this chapter focuses on the typical adjustments that most people experience as part of redefining and updating their relationship with food and eating behaviour. These adjustments happen in different domains – psychological, behavioural and environmental. Psychological adjustments include redefining your relationship with food, mourning the loss of food, finding alternative sources of enjoyment and finding a healthy balance. Behavioural adjustments involve managing your new eating experience and responses, eating mindfully and eating regularly despite not feeling hungry. Environmental adjustments include managing eating in social situations, at home and at work.

The second part of the chapter focuses on binge eating/loss-of-control eating and grazing eating patterns. It is important to discuss these specific eating patterns because if they continue to be a problem or re-emerge following surgery, they can affect how much weight someone loses, as well as their psychological health and quality of life. Focusing on the ways in which you can make positive adjustments should prevent (or at least reduce the risk) of some of these high-risk eating behaviours returning or emerging.

Adjusting your psychological relationship with food

Redefining how you view food

Bariatric surgery can sometimes act as a "reset" button – it creates a clean break from a previous pattern of eating. The meaning of food often changes to focus on nutrition and health, not being on a diet. The prescribed post-operative texture progression plan often seems to break the connection with old eating patterns and creates an opportunity for a new beginning.

My relationship with food is dramatically different – prior to the surgery, food was in abundance, it was a celebration, it was reward, it was comfort, it was a reaction to emotions and social situations. And now it is purely driven by physical need – I have hunger and I have to eat for health. There is no question that the celebratory aspect of eating has completely gone and you have to grieve for it. You don't really eat for pleasure, you eat for need.

AM, 6 months post sleeve

Before surgery, people often describe their eating as feeling "out of control". After surgery, they often feel more in control of their eating, but this is only maintained if they proactively work at making helpful choices and decisions along the way.

I don't have that sense of not being able to stop when I start eating now. It has completely changed. I can opt for healthier choices now. When you've done so much and come so far, you don't want to undo it all and go back. If I'm in the shop buying a sandwich I'll look at several different options and find a balance between one that I like but that's not as bad as the worst one.

JT, 18 months post bypass who used to binge eat prior to surgery

After bariatric surgery, people often feel more capable of influencing their behaviour because they have a tool to work with which gives them physical feedback rather than just having to rely on their own internal resources. This seems to make a huge difference to people's confidence in their ability to make changes. However, it's also important that you explicitly acknowledge your contribution in making the tool of surgery work. It is a partnership. The eating and physical activity behaviours that you choose to put in place can really help to maintain that feeling of being in control.

Finding a middle ground – "good enough, not perfect"

Eating choices after surgery should be based around eating to improve and maintain your health – this can still be enjoyable! This includes allowing yourself to have occasional treats (obviously with limits on the amount and frequency) as part of developing a healthy relationship with food.

After surgery, people often find that the internal debates and arguments that they have about food are much quieter and less noticeable.

I now feel back in control. I've started to lose weight so I feel like a happier person. My headspace is vastly improved for not having to focus every minute of every day on what shall I eat and that internal battle between eating and not eating. My head is much less noisy because I'm in a place where I am not dictated to by food. I feel that I can make choices now. The power has gone from food and I hope it stays that way.

VS, 2 years post bypass

As you can see from the quote above, there is a shift from feeling deprived and focusing on foods that are not "allowed", and there is a sense of liberation that arises as a result.

There's no sense of being deprived anymore – I'm out of that dieting mindset. I can have small amounts of what I want and that feels great.

AM, 6 months post sleeve

This style of eating involves not depriving yourself and not overindulging either. We are looking for a middle ground between these positions.

It is ironic that moving away from dieting and dieting rules often tends to help people make long-term changes and lose weight!

Loss of food and having to cope with difficult emotions

For those people who have previously relied on food to manage or suppress their emotions, the initial period following surgery can be challenging when they experience emotions and aren't able to use food to manage them. Others may find that they experience emotions that they haven't previously allowed themselves to feel – food has been a protective blanket. There can be a sense of mourning over the loss of food as it has sometimes been the main support or consistent friend that someone has had throughout their life.

It was like everything just hit me all at once because I'd lost food. It was like it was gone and that was all I had growing up. Every traumatic or upsetting situation, the fix was food so when that was gone, it was like food had blocked everything before and someone's just punched you right in the face. The first time it happened, it hit hard. I was kind of like 'what do I do now?' Most of the time now I can handle those difficult times and I'm getting better at dealing with them – I can be upset without needing to escape from it or I can feel it coming on and distract myself and let it pass over.

JT, 9 months post sleeve, previously used food to block out feelings

There were a couple of times shortly after surgery when I felt really panicked and was thinking 'What do I do instead?' There was definitely a need to do something to manage how I was feeling. One thing I've noticed more recently is that alcohol can act as that. There is still that need to have that kind of release and I just have to try to find something that's safe and healthy.

ER, 15 months post bypass

This is a temporary stage and will get easier over time. It takes time to build up your resilience and confidence in your ability to manage emotions. It might feel difficult, but it will be worthwhile. You can use some of the strategies outlined in Chapter 3 to help you cope with difficult or new emotions without using food as a coping strategy.

Reduced enjoyment from food

Some people may have previously derived a lot of pleasure and enjoyment from eating, and this may no longer be the case after surgery. They can go through a process of grieving for food because they miss the role that it previously played in their lives and the enjoyment that they got from it.

Food makes me feel good. It takes away almost everything. It gives me intense pleasure. I feel calm and soothed. I love nothing more than I love food. Even now I still have that love . . . I think that part of that relationship is still there. Having the physical help makes a difference because I can't eat as much. I do try to control my love for food too. I haven't found anything to take its place and that is part of the trouble. It is a loss. I really grieved for the pleasure that I used to have. I have to be really focused on what I am eating and when . . . if I lose that control, that other part of me creeps back in. My head is the problem part . . . I am fighting all the time to tell myself that food doesn't mean more to me than sustenance.

GM, 5 years post bypass

This grieving process is more likely to happen in the early stages after surgery when the loss of food is felt most profoundly. This often changes over time, especially when people are able to feel the benefits and rewards of the weight loss. These benefits often mean that people don't need to rely on food in the same way as before.

Others find that their relationship with food can change dramatically during these early days from pleasure to dislike/disinterest. They have to switch into an alien mindset of pushing themselves to eat because it is no longer enjoyable.

> Food was not my friend. I became very impatient and started to resent food. I resented the effort and thought and planning that had to go into food. Nothing came easy, it was an effort. But I worked through it and being aware of the issue is the important bit.
>
> AM, 6 months post sleeve

> When I saw the surgeon about three months after my operation, he told me that I needed to start eating a bit more and start eating more solid foods. I didn't enjoy food and had to push myself to eat it. There was nothing that I was enjoying taste-wise . . . for the first time in my whole life I wasn't interested in food and it didn't bother me whether I ate or not.
>
> AE, 9 months post bypass

It can be a very strange and disconcerting experience when people find that the urge to eat has disappeared, and that they have to force themselves to eat despite not feeling hungry. There are changes to taste buds and sense of smell that may occur (particularly after a bypass), which can also affect people's experiences of eating. This does tend to be a temporary phase, but it can lead to problems with not eating enough to maintain health or losing weight too quickly. It is important to discuss this with your bariatric team, as they will be able to offer ideas and strategies to support you.

Finding other sources of pleasure and enjoyment

As you may not get as much enjoyment out of food, it is important to think about other things that make you feel good or that you enjoy. Many people find that they can capitalise on their weight loss to do things that were previously not possible. This in itself can help reduce the focus and reliance on food that some people previously had, as the quotations below highlight.

Because I've got my mobility back, food isn't as important to me. I don't have the same focus on eating to make myself feel better. I've got other options available like taking the dog for a walk etc.

PK, 9 months post sleeve

I've got so much energy now that I didn't have before. It is so much easier to do things that make me feel good. I've noticed that I'm much more outward-looking than I used to be before my surgery when I used to stay at home and eat in the evenings. Now, I want to try doing new things and do the things that I felt I couldn't do before. I don't need to eat in the way that I did before because I've got other things I want to do.

ER, 18 months post bypass

Adjusting your eating behaviours

Following surgery there are eating changes and adjustments that will help you re-educate your digestive system after bariatric surgery. The digestive system is radically altered as a result of the surgery – the stomach is significantly smaller, portion sizes will be much smaller and there will be some foods that will be difficult to tolerate (these vary between people).

It is helpful to think about the first six months after surgery as a learning process where you get to know your new stomach, how it works and what you need to do to keep it functioning in a way that is consistent with your weight loss goals. Your body will give you feedback if you tune into it. There are some key areas that you will need to focus your learning on:

- Adjusting your portion sizes
- Making the best choices for your stomach/body
- Identifying foods that do and don't work for you.

As mentioned previously, it's very important to get these foundations in place early on, as the research shows that the different weight loss trajectories start to emerge around six months after surgery.

Some other important changes to help you adjust to your new eating pattern are outlined below.

Planning ahead

It is important to make sure that you plan your eating. Some people use a meal plan for the week and then base their shopping (and shopping list) around this. If you plan your meals and your shopping then it is much more likely that you will have the right foods around you, and this will help you stay on track.

This active planning approach will help you use your "thinking brain" when making decisions about food, not your "emotional brain". This means that you are doing the brainwork before the event!

Monitoring your eating and weight

Keeping track of your eating and weight is one of the best ways of maintaining a sense of control. Knowledge is power, so if you have access to the right information then you can make modifications or relax knowing that you are on track.

Using your updated 'bariatric eyes and stomach'

Sometimes people describe how "their eyes are still bigger than their belly" after surgery, and so they make decisions about their portion sizes based on old behaviour patterns. Make active decisions about your portion sizes using bariatric guidance. This involves making an active decision about when to stop eating – don't push it. Remind yourself that it is okay to leave food.

Eating slowly and mindfully

One of the main reasons people may struggle with their eating after surgery is that they are eating too quickly and/or not chewing their food enough. Make sure that you are eating slowly and mindfully. This can also help you to feel satisfied and full after eating a small portion of food. It takes the brain a while to register that you are full, so the slower you eat the more chance you have of recognising this point. Eating slowly and mindfully can also help you to get the maximum pleasure out of a small amount of food.

- Eat mindfully (you can use the exercise in Chapter 23).
- Time yourself – about 20 minutes for a meal.
- Count the number of times you chew before you swallow – you are aiming for about 20 or as close to this number as possible.
- Put your knife and fork down in between mouthfuls.
- Pace yourself with someone who is a slow eater.
- Make an active decision about eating your last mouthful – this is because people often describe experiencing pain or regurgitation when they have eaten one mouthful too many.

Eating regularly without hunger signals

Another adjustment people have to make after surgery is getting into a pattern of eating regularly despite not feeling hungry. Sometimes people feel relief that they no longer have to struggle with feeling hungry, and this means that they sometimes skip meals and don't eat enough to maintain their health. If you skip meals and don't eat for many hours, you may experience nausea, and this can sometimes put people off eating again – another vicious cycle!

What are the consequences of not eating regularly? One of the consequences is low blood sugar, which causes problems with headaches, concentration and lethargy (in severe cases, it can cause seizures and loss of consciousness). In addition, there is a higher risk of nutritional deficiencies. Skipping meals also contributes to problems with constipation. In the longer term, eating regular meals will help people regulate their energy intake to prevent over eating and aid better food choices. Hunger causes people to choose poor nutritional quality foods which are more likely to contribute towards weight gain. Also, individuals who consume more calories later in the day have less time to be active to burn off these extra calories.

It can feel "wrong" to eat when not feeling hungry as this breaks many of the dieting rules that people have previously followed. However, the hunger signals are disrupted after bariatric surgery, so it is important to set regular times to eat and plan what you are going to eat.

Recognising satiety

Following bariatric surgery, there are also changes in the hormones that make you feel full or satiated after eating. Most people describe feeling full after eating very small amounts of food. It is important to tune in and respect these signals rather than pushing the limits of what you can eat (this could potentially stretch your stomach pouch over time).

In this stage, you are trying to learn and recalibrate the relationship between your portion sizes and satiety. Portion sizes are likely to be a great deal smaller after surgery, and it takes a while to learn how little food is needed before you feel satisfied or full. Sometimes people still end up putting too much food on their plate, and this can either overface them (therefore putting them off eating), or it means they are tempted and eat more than they need.

Coping with fear of vomiting and avoidance of certain foods and textures

Occasionally, people may have repeated experiences of vomiting or pain after eating certain foods, and this can lead to anxiety and avoidance and can develop into a food aversion. The body and the brain learn to make negative associations between eating the specific food(s) and the consequences (pain/vomiting). This is a problem because it puts you at risk of having an incomplete diet, and it restricts people's lives. It can also lead to weight regain as people tend to shift towards having a softer diet or having high-calorie foods such as chocolate or crisps which are often eaten without causing problems.

It would be helpful to speak to the dietitian in your bariatric service to see whether they can advise you about different ways of preparing or eating those specific foods. It is possible that you tried to move onto the next stage of texture progression too quickly (this varies between people), so you may need to take a step back to a soft or even liquid phase before trying those foods again.

If all these options have been explored then it's time to focus on building your confidence so that you (and your new stomach) can learn to tolerate those foods and no longer need to avoid them.

> I remember those early months and the difficulties shifting phases from liquids to purees . . . I just couldn't do it. That was a bit of a crisis for me. I had to be brave and started to move into more solid foods and nothing awful happened.
>
> AM, 8 months post surgery

How to deal with this?

You can build up your confidence in eating certain foods by working out a step-by-step approach to facing your problem foods. Think of it as a ladder with each rung being a small step towards building up your confidence. This is called graded exposure – it's the same approach as helping someone with a phobia. For example, a post-op woman who was struggling to get back onto solid foods because she was anxious about vomiting used the following ladder:

Step 1 – Thin/smooth soups

Step 2 – Chunky or half-blended soups

Step 3 – Fish or slow-cooked stew made with vegetables, potatoes and beans

Step 4 – Introduce minced meat into regime via dishes such as shepherd's pie/bolognaise-style sauce

(continued)

(continued)

> Step 5 – Casserole/slow-cook meals with bigger chunks of meat or fish
>
> Step 6 – Casserole/slow-cook meals with small chunks of meat but draining out the sauce before eating.

Your bariatric team will be able to help you work out your own graded exposure food ladder.

Adjusting and managing your environment

Social eating

People sometimes assume that they will no longer be able to eat out in restaurants after having bariatric surgery. This can make people worry that their friendships and relationships will suffer because they can no longer participate in the same way as before surgery. However, you CAN eat out socially and visit restaurants as long as you make wise decisions. It is often better to wait until you have got through the texture progression diet to try eating out.

- Plan ahead – check menus online and work out what might be most suitable.
- Make requests in restaurants – be assertive, specify what you would like. Some people may choose to let the restaurant know that they have had surgery (it is your choice if you specify bariatric) and that you are limited to certain foods/portion sizes.
- Learn how to order wisely for yourself as highlighted below.
- Often people may choose to order starters as a main course (you could even have two starters – one as a starter and then the other for your main course).

I've learned to order food in a certain way that works for me – you just have to come up with strategies. I order salad as a starter and fish for a main course without any side dishes and that works really well for me.

PM, 10 months post surgery

Sometimes people worry that others will focus on their eating if they know that they have had bariatric surgery. You may find that others question why you are only eating such small amounts or leaving food. It can be helpful to prepare some responses in advance for these scenarios so that you don't have to think on the spot. Of course, your response is going to differ depending on whether you want to tell others that you have had bariatric surgery. If you are happy to tell people then you can simply say, "This is the amount of food I have been advised to eat after my surgery" or "Since my surgery, it's really important for me to notice when I feel full as otherwise I could end up being ill". If you prefer not to tell others about your surgery then you could state that "I'm trying to make some changes to my eating and think more carefully about my portion sizes" or "I'd rather leave food than feel that I have eaten too much – that works better for me".

If your social life previously revolved around eating out, then this is an opportunity to think about other ways of spending time with friends whilst you are building up your confidence. It is helpful to focus on planning and doing other things with people, for example, going to the cinema, going for a walk, going to a gallery and so on. We tend to get stuck in a rut in terms of our social activities, so this can be a positive opportunity to spend time together doing different things.

Socialising may involve managing your alcohol intake. Alcohol is generally to be avoided after bariatric surgery, partly because of the empty calories that it contains, but more importantly because of the evidence that there is an increased risk of developing alcohol dependency problems (for those who have had gastric bypass surgery). If you drink alcohol, you are likely to become intoxicated very quickly from a small amount of alcohol, and it remains in your blood stream for a longer period of time.

Eating at home

There are some basics to get in place when eating meals at home.

- Put your meal on a plate instead of grazing. Sometimes people may start to feel overfaced by meals as they can only each very small amounts and this can lead to a "grazing" pattern of eating to avoid that feeling. It's important to get into the habit of having a meal because that is part of developing a healthy relationship with food, and also the grazing pattern can be problematic.

- Sit down to eat at the table. Similarly to above, sometimes people may avoid eating and so eat whilst doing other things to reduce the amount of attention they have to pay to it. Again, this is a problematic habit because it can lead to people not paying attention to what they are eating and how they are eating. This leaves people vulnerable to making inappropriate food choices or eating too quickly and therefore experiencing pain/regurgitation.

Managing your work environment

You will also need to think about how you manage your eating in your work environment – it sometimes gets in the way and causes problems! For example, if you work in a very busy environment with lots of time pressure, you could end up skipping meals or not drinking enough water. You will need to negotiate regular breaks or find ways of reminding yourself to take a break.

It can also be challenging if you work in an environment where chocolate/biscuits and cake are usually around – this means you need to be extra vigilant. Depending on your work set-up, you could suggest either moving them to a different part of the office where they are less visible, or you could see if people are interested in swapping them for another type of food. Alternatively, it may be up to you to change your response, and so limit the number of times you walk past them. Think about some key phrases you can use to decline them if they are offered to you, as well.

It can really help to plan what, how and where you are going to eat at work. By focusing on this, the other challenges outlined above shouldn't be such an issue. If you take food with you to work and plan what time you are going to have it then you are in control!

Challenges and pitfalls to negotiate

In this section, we will focus on two high-risk eating behaviours (loss-of-control eating and graze eating) that are associated with poorer weight loss and/or weight regain.

Loss-of-control eating

As we discussed earlier in the book, a significant number of people struggle with binge eating patterns prior to surgery. After surgery, people do not binge in the same way because they are unable to eat such large quantities of food. Having said that, binge eating can still be a problem: it just looks slightly different. The loss-of-control or out-of-control feeling that was connected with binge eating before surgery may continue. That is why this pattern of eating is called "loss-of-control eating" after surgery.

What is loss-of-control eating?

A questionnaire was developed to tap into the main behaviours associated with loss-of-control eating (Blomquist et al. 2014). People are asked to record how many times in the past 28 days certain behaviours have occurred. These include:

- giving in to impulses to eat
- not being able to stop eating when started
- feeling helpless and unable to control food urges
- making a decision before eating not to control what you are going to eat
- going out of your way to get food that you crave
- keeping eating even though you felt you should stop.

Loss-of-control eating tends not to be an immediate problem after surgery but often re-emerges after a few months. A research study found that this pattern starts to emerge about six months following surgery, and the number of people experiencing it increases over time from 31% at six months to 39% at two years. Those people who experience this type of eating lose less weight over time (White et al. 2010). A study which reviewed most of the research done found that 14 of the 15 studies confirmed the negative effects of post-op binge eating/loss-of-control eating on weight loss (Meany et al. 2014).

Why is loss-of-control eating still an issue? The triggers that previously affected people's emotional responses may remain after surgery (or can recur). If someone hasn't developed other ways of coping then it is understandable that eating would remain their first port of call. It is very important to be aware of this pattern early on and work towards nipping it in the bud as soon as possible.

Strategies

- Work at regaining a sense of control. Loss-of-control eating is often more likely to happen or recur when other aspects of life have led to a feeling of being out of control. This is often during periods of heightened stress or when there are life changes. There are two different places where you can focus – first, there may be some things that you need to do to regain a sense of control over your wider life, for example, distinguishing between areas that you can and cannot influence, and then problem-solving around the former. Second, regaining a sense of control over your eating – it is helpful to focus on making small changes to re-establish the foundations rather than simply try to eliminate binge eating or loss-of-control eating episodes. These changes include tracking your eating, planning your meals and your shopping, planning appropriate foods to take out with you and talking to others about how you are trying to actively manage your eating. It is also helpful to think back to previous times when you have managed to regain a sense of control – what worked for you then?

- Identifying triggers and responding differently to them. What has led to you feeling this way? Is this something that is within your control or that you can influence? If so, use your problem-solving skills to think about any other options that might help you deal with the actual problem.
- Write down how you are feeling/name these emotions. You can destroy what you have written afterwards if you are concerned that someone may find it.
- Explore what happens to your emotions. Build up your tolerance to them. Learn that you can experience emotions without necessarily having to respond to them.
- Check to see if you have the basics in place. Plan meals and eat regularly. These are really important blocks to stop people slipping back into old habits. Also, if you eat regularly, you are more likely to respond to things rationally and less emotionally.
- Seek support.
- If you have a history of mental health problems then it is also important to check that your mental health hasn't changed, destabilised or deteriorated, as this could be another reason why your eating has changed. There is more information about this in Chapter 8, but it is important to mention that you should seek help as soon as possible.

Grazing

There has recently been more focus on graze eating (also known as "picking and nibbling") after bariatric surgery as it is associated with poorer weight loss outcomes. It appears that people who had difficulties with binge eating before surgery are at risk of converting to a grazing pattern following surgery, and this is equally problematic (Colles et al. 2008). This might be because it is easier to graze with a smaller stomach than binge eat. The reliance on food just shifts in its presentation.

How is grazing defined?

Grazing is defined as unplanned, mindless/absent-minded eating and continuous food consumption (Zunker et al. 2012). It is the process of continuously picking at food without ever feeling full or satisfied.

The food helps with the boredom because it helps the time pass by. Eating is something you can do again 30 minutes later. It's a mechanical thing. Like being a robot . . . and a cycle I keep repeating. I'd feel terrible at the end of the day. It's a dark cycle.

AC, 2 years post-op bypass, regained 20kg

A study found that frequent grazing is associated with weight regain. People who reported grazing at least two times per week had greater weight regain and less weight loss (Kofman et al. 2010). Some people find that their grazing feels compulsive and difficult to control, and is sometimes associated with trying to manage feelings of anxiety. Another study (Goodpaster et al. 2015) found that those people who graze experience higher levels of distress and are generally more anxious and depressed.

It's important to distinguish between "little and often" eating patterns that are helpful and planned and grazing which is characterised by going from snack to snack in an unplanned, distracted manner and is often emotionally driven.

Strategies to manage grazing

- Increasing your awareness and making conscious choices/decisions
- Questioning "Does this look like a meal?"
- Questioning "How long was it since you last ate?" – create a clear gap
- Managing your food environment to set limitations
- Evaluating the foods you graze on. Are there any particular meanings or memories attached?

Summary

Adjusting your eating and your relationship with food after surgery takes time. It is an ongoing process and different issues will crop up at different time points during your journey. Making these adjustments won't just occur overnight. There may be times where you slip back into old habits and have to refocus your attention. It is important to get a balance between recognising how far you have come alongside which old habits you need to keep an eye out for and what you need to keep working on.

References

Blomquist, K.K., et al., 2014. Development and validation of the Eating Loss of Control Scale. *Psychological Assessment*, 26 (1), 77–89 doi:10.103a0034729.

Colles, S.L., et al., 2008. Grazing and loss of control related to eating: two high-risk factors following bariatric surgery. *Obesity*, 16 (3), 615–22.

Goodpaster, K. et al., 2015. Grazing eating among bariatric surgery candidates: prevalence and psychosocial correlates. *Surgery for Obesity and Related Diseases*, 11 (6), S50–S51.

Kofman, M.D., et al., 2010. Maladaptive eating patterns, quality of life, and weight outcomes following gastric bypass: results of an internet survey. *Obesity*, 18 (10), 1938–1943.

Meany, G., et al., 2014. Binge eating, binge eating disorder and loss of control eating: effects on weight outcomes after bariatric surgery. *European Eating Disorders Review*, 22 (2), 87–91.

White, M.A. et al., 2010. Loss of control over eating predicts outcomes in bariatric surgery: a prospective 24-month follow up study. *Journal of Clinical Psychiatry*, 71 (2), 175–184.

Zunker, C., et al., 2012. Eating behaviors post-bariatric surgery: a qualitative study of grazing. Obesity surgery, 22 (8), 1225–31.

Chapter 8

Improving psychological wellbeing and managing psychological pitfalls after surgery

We often focus on weight loss as the main measure of success after bariatric surgery, but it is also important to consider the impact of bariatric surgery on how you feel emotionally. Weight loss after surgery is positive, but it can bring unanticipated adjustments and changes. Bariatric surgery is a psychological intervention, as well as a weight loss intervention.

Earlier in the book, we discussed how bariatric surgery is a fantastic opportunity to make changes, but it also creates psychological challenges. It can sometimes be difficult to anticipate or truly appreciate how these changes will feel until after surgery has happened – it can take the most confident and well-prepared people by surprise. We want to tip the balance in the right direction so that you experience more positives than challenges!

The first part of this chapter focuses on ways to enhance psychological wellbeing through making the most of the psychological opportunity that bariatric surgery presents. Surgery becomes a springboard for making changes to how you feel about yourself and the opportunities you engage with in your wider life.

The second part of the chapter focuses on finding ways of managing some of the psychological pitfalls that have been shown to lead to poor weight loss and can leave people feeling very distressed and unhappy.

These difficulties can arise at any point after surgery, but in my experience, they tend to either arise fairly soon after surgery or when weight loss is slowing or has stopped. Psychological difficulties can emerge after surgery if food has been someone's main coping mechanism and they have not found other ways of coping. Also, rapid weight loss can lead to feelings of vulnerability for some people. In the longer term, difficulties can re-emerge when the excitement of surgery has worn off and weight loss has slowed or stopped. Psychological improvements are often dependent on weight loss, and this can leave people vulnerable to emotional changes when their loss slows or stops. This is one of the reasons why it's important to develop strategies to manage emotional health, so that people are not completely reliant on weight loss.

Building confidence and embracing new opportunities: using surgery and weight loss as a springboard

Many people find that their confidence generally improves after surgery. Weight problems are often closely linked with low confidence, so as someone starts to lose weight, they often notice that their confidence starts to improve. However, this can also create a challenge for some people as their previous weight issues may have created a plausible reason for not doing things in the past. The fact that their weight is no longer a reason for not doing something can create anxiety. For example, one woman had stayed in the same job for years and had avoided going for promotion opportunities because of her worries about how she thought other people judged her weight. As she lost weight, she felt pressure to apply for promotions because her original reason for not applying was no longer valid.

If you have avoided doing things for a long time, it is understandable that your confidence in your ability to manage these things might be low. People sometimes find that they need to develop new skills because they have avoided certain situations before.

Sometimes weight loss and confidence can become too closely intertwined so that as you lose weight, confidence improves, and if you gain weight, confidence decreases. It is important not to be completely reliant on weight loss to influence your confidence as this leaves you less vulnerable to having dips when your weight loss slows and stops.

People have often experienced stigma and judgement because of their weight, and this may have affected their self-esteem. It affects how people feel about themselves (and how they think others view them). For some, this means that they start to avoid situations because they don't want to be exposed to potential judgement. This avoidance might reduce their anxiety in the short term because they don't have to face a situation that they are scared about, but it also perpetuates low confidence. Life shuts down for people. This avoidance means that they deny themselves the opportunity to be reminded about what they are good at or what they can do. Weight loss can be the start of trying to improve your confidence and self-esteem.

Behaviours associated with low confidence and self-esteem

- Avoiding situations
- Isolating self
- Deferring to others
- Apologising
- Putting yourself down (including joking at your own expense).

Thought patterns associated with low confidence and self-esteem

- Making negative predictions about your competence/effectiveness
- Mindreading by making negative predictions about how others will respond to or judge you
- Criticising yourself.

The patterns of thinking and behaviour that are signs of low self-esteem and poor confidence actually reinforce these feelings.

For example, if someone makes negative predictions about being harassed and bullied by people if they were to go out, then it is likely that they will avoid going out. As a result of avoiding the situation, they never get to find out that either their predictions didn't materialise or that they do have the skills to cope with the situation. Choices and decisions start to be based on their anxiety and avoidance rather than what they actually want to do.

- What are some of the things you may not have been able to do previously or may not have allowed yourself to do?
- Are there things that you still want to do where you feel your confidence is stopping you or holding you back?

It might also be useful to ask people you are close to whether they feel that your weight/confidence has stopped you from doing certain things,

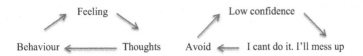

Figure 8.1 Vicious cycle of low self-esteem

too. They may have a different perspective and be able to spot things that you are no longer aware of.

The following strategies will help you to find more helpful thinking patterns and behaviours to build your confidence.

Building blocks to facilitate adjustment and wellbeing

Building up confidence step-by-step – approaching, not avoiding

If there are things that you would like to do but feel worried or frightened about trying, try to work out a step-by-step approach to building your confidence. This involves pushing yourself out of your comfort zone but taking small steps to achieve your ultimate goal or achieving the things you want to be able to. The more you do it, the easier it becomes.

You might want to picture this as a ladder, with your goal at the top of the ladder and each rung as a step towards it. When you are working out what goes on each rung of the ladder, it helps to identify things that push you out of your comfort zone but not so much that you feel completely overwhelmed. The idea is to move onto the next rung of the ladder once you feel that you can confidently manage the rung that you are currently on.

The example below is of a confidence ladder for a woman who was frightened of being around people because she predicted that they would make negative comments about her weight. She therefore used to spend a lot of time indoors. This meant that her activity levels were low, and she was more prone to emotional eating when she was indoors.

Going to the cinema

Going for a meal with friend

Staying for a coffee in a shop

Going to library to ask about courses

Shopping in town centre

Shopping in a larger shop

Walking to the nearest shop

Walking to the end of the road

Figure 8.2 Example of a confidence ladder

Remember that as you push yourself to try things you haven't done before, it's completely natural to feel some anxiety – it will pass. Think back to other things you might have been scared about doing for the first time and how these became natural and automatic over time. For example, after passing their driving test, most people are anxious and apprehensive about driving by themselves for the first time. As you drive more frequently, your confidence builds, and it becomes automatic – you no longer think about it as an anxiety-provoking event!

Build your confidence by changing your internal conversation

We tend not to pay much attention to our internal conversations and how these affect us when we are planning to try something new. The way you view a situation, and the type of predictions you make about it, can either block you or encourage you.

Below are some questions you can use to encourage yourself to approach situations with confidence:

- How would you encourage a friend in a similar situation? Are you saying the same things to yourself or something different?
- What's the worst that could happen? How likely is it that the worst *will* happen and that the worst *won't* happen? What is your evidence?
- Think about the predictions that you have previously made and how accurate they have been. What does this tell you? It can be useful to write out beforehand what you predict and anticipate will happen in the situation you are approaching, and then review this afterwards. This is one way of checking out how accurate your predictions are.

Finding your internal supporter and quietening the "internal bully"

We are often our own worst critic and speak to ourselves in a way that we would never speak to anyone else. We often tend to bully ourselves and focus only on our shortcomings and mistakes and magnify them. Over time, we have often trained our brains to pay far more attention to what we do "wrong" than what we do well. This means that our attention becomes biased towards the negative, therefore lowering our self-esteem and confidence. As a result of focusing on our perceived failings, our motivation to make changes also suffers. Why bother trying when you predict you won't be able to manage it or succeed? It is highly likely that the problem is your confidence, not your competence. In order to build confidence, we need to give equal or fair attention to what we are doing well in addition to what we need to work on.

People sometimes believe that being self-critical is a way of holding themselves accountable, and that it is only by "shouting" or berating themselves that they will become motivated and get on track. However, if you step back and think about it, does this actually work? If you recall your early years at school, which teachers did you do your best work for – those that were critical or those that were encouraging?

Give yourself credit for what you are doing well

The aim is to help you notice improvements and changes but also identify areas of tension or struggle that you can focus your effort and energy on resolving.

It is really important to learn how to shift your attention to what you are achieving and doing well. Try to pay attention and regularly record some of the things that you can now do that you were unable to manage before, for example, putting socks on/walking further/crossing your legs/ fastening car seatbelt easier. You could look back at your pre-surgery photos and clothes as an objective record of how far you have come.

Focusing on yourself

There is often a stark discrepancy between how people treat themselves compared to how they treat other people. This manifests itself in different ways, for example, the way you speak or relate to others (in comparison to yourself), the amount of time you might dedicate to them, the support you give them and the way you praise them when they have achieved something.

It is important to make sure that you are putting enough time and effort into your post-surgery experience to make it work. People who are distracted and who spend a lot of time caring and putting others before themselves tend not to do so well – they just don't have the time to do what is required.

For example, one woman found that she had to unexpectedly take on a lot of caring responsibilities after her surgery. This meant that she had no time to plan her eating or eat regularly because she was caring for everyone else. The fact that she was not losing as much weight as expected after surgery made her feel like a failure as well as feeling angry with others for jeopardising her opportunity. Obviously, there are times when there are unexpected challenges and demands in life, but working out your minimum non-negotiable requirements for yourself is important. This might include making sure that you have enough time to do a weekly shop, making sure you have appropriate emergency snacks to carry with you and that you have time to prepare quick meals. Sometimes people feel that it is "wrong" to dedicate time and attention to themselves. Just because something feels "wrong", it doesn't necessarily mean it is – there is a big difference between something being unfamiliar and something being wrong. Try asking yourself why you wouldn't deserve to be treated like others.

Some of these changes which involve treating yourself more fairly and equally can create ripples in relationship dynamics. It can take time for others to get used to a newly assertive you and adjust to the fact that you may be less available to do things for them. This can create difficult and uncomfortable feelings, and you may be tempted to revert to old patterns. Stick with it and allow others time to adjust.

Accepting positive feedback – responding to compliments

As you start to lose weight, you may receive more compliments from others. Whilst this can be a very positive experience, it can sometimes be difficult for people to know how to react or respond. This is particularly the case for people whose self-esteem is low who often have a habit of dismissing compliments. The problem with dismissing compliments is that the person never gets to fully process or take on board this positive feedback, and their confidence remains low. It's as though they don't allow the positive feedback to stay in their brain for long enough, unlike negative feedback which tends to be focused on and scrutinised in great depth.

> It was difficult to know what to do or say when people complimented me after surgery – I just felt really embarrassed by it because I hadn't really had that experience before. I just didn't know what to say back or how to move the conversation on. I eventually learned to just say 'thank you' and that worked ok.
>
> HB, 12 months post sleeve gastrectomy

> People commented on my weight a lot more afterwards and I took it really badly. People would say, 'Oh my god, you look really amazing' and I'd snap back, 'What, because I looked such a state before?' And they would say, 'No, it's just a compliment'. I was just so sensitive to it.
>
> NR, 4 years post bypass

Various strategies for responding to compliments include:

- Just say, "Thank you" and smile.
- Acknowledge the compliment by saying, "That's kind of you to say".
- Ask them a question to refocus their attention.

Some people also describe feeling fraudulent when accepting compliments about their weight loss, for a couple of reasons. One is when someone hasn't disclosed that they have bariatric surgery, and they find that they are getting lots of positive feedback. They can feel guilty for taking credit for something without disclosing the complete picture. Remember you have a choice about how much information you choose to share with people. We all have aspects of our lives that we choose to keep private.

Adjusting to no longer feeling stigmatised

People often describe feeling that they "fit in" better, and that they don't feel as judged as a result of losing weight after bariatric surgery. There are obviously some positive aspects to feeling this way, but it can also be challenging as it may trigger resentment about how they were previously treated. These experiences of being treated better and/or differently by others just because their weight has changed can lead to feelings of irritation and anger. It can be a painful glimpse of how shallow and superficial others can be when they treat you with more interest and respect simply because your weight has changed. It's also worth bearing in mind that people may treat you differently because they have noticed a change in your confidence and willingness to engage with them, too.

Feeling self-conscious – visible and noticeable

Some people feel proud of their weight loss and want others to notice and pay attention. However, for others it can feel uncomfortable being the centre of attention with the spotlight firmly fixed on your weight loss. This can be particularly awkward if you preferred to be in the background before. Often people have learned to cope with these experiences by avoiding situations or remaining in the background in order to feel less noticeable and safe.

It is helpful to be prepared for the fact that your weight loss (and eating) is likely to be commented upon by people you know as well as strangers.

> At first when you are losing weight, people don't know if you are just ill . . . the bigger friends I've had seem to be jealous about my weight loss but other people are positive.
>
> PK, 12 months post bypass

> Your weight and what people see you eat will be commented on. At first it was difficult to deal with the positive and negative comments about my weight loss – you will be open season for everyone to comment on what you look like and they are completely oblivious to how it makes you feel. It was not just the comments on my physical appearance but people obsessing about what I was eating because they are so interested. I found the compliments difficult to know how to deal with. And the negative comments have been difficult too . . . I've been called 'too skinny' and told 'you're taking this too far' and I didn't know how to deal with it. I've come up with a strategy so if someone gives me a compliment I just say, 'Thank you, that's so kind – I feel great' and if they say something negative I say, 'I've never felt better' and they can't argue with that! You just have to recognise that there will be lots of compliments coming your way and just accept them. When you get any negative feedback just reassure them that you are ok.
>
> AM, 10 months post bypass

As people lose weight, they can feel increasingly visible or noticeable to others, and this can sometimes lead to feeling more vulnerable in the outside world. In my experience, this can be a particular challenge for those people who have had difficult and abusive experiences earlier in life – this may include sexual abuse but also includes bullying and harassment. This is discussed in more detail in Chapter 10, which focuses on body image.

Psychological problems

Most people find that after bariatric surgery, their mental health and psychological wellbeing improve. However, it would be wrong not to highlight some of the mental health difficulties that can occur after surgery which can create serious problems. These are rare events, but you need to be aware of them so that if they arise you can seek help quickly.

Depression

Rates of depression following surgery improve significantly – a recent study found that 45% of people were depressed before surgery and this dropped to 12% after surgery. There is some evidence that for a sub-group of people who have bariatric surgery, rates of depression start to creep up again as time after surgery increases (White et al. 2015). For example, one study found that a particular high-risk period for depression returning is between six to 12 months following surgery, which is when the "honeymoon period" ends (Ivezaj and Grilo 2015). People who become depressed after bariatric surgery are at risk of losing less weight, and depression is obviously a debilitating and distressing condition to live with.

Why do people get depressed after bariatric surgery?

Depression is often a problem that recurs. If someone has had an episode of depression previously, they are at greater risk of having a further episode of depression. As there are higher rates of depression amongst people seeking bariatric surgery, it is logical that some people will experience depression again because of their history. Obviously, bariatric surgery doesn't prevent stressful or difficult life events happening, and these can trigger depression. Furthermore, bariatric surgery itself can be challenging and can therefore trigger depression.

Causes of depression related to bariatric surgery include:

- complications and difficulties following surgery requiring hospital admissions
- difficulties managing the post-op diet
- unmet expectations of weight loss and the changes that weight loss may lead to in your life
- realising that some problems still remain
- not being able to use food to self-medicate
- medication not working effectively
- excess skin/body image issues
- relationship changes.

What are the symptoms of depression?

The main symptoms of depression are:
   Psychological symptoms

- Feeling continuously low in mood
- Feeling tearful

- Feeling hopeless and helpless
- Feeling irritable and intolerant of others
- Lacking in motivation
- Finding it difficult to make decisions
- Not getting any enjoyment out of life
- Feeling anxious or worried
- Having suicidal thoughts.

Physical symptoms

- Lack of energy
- Low sex drive or libido
- Disturbed sleep
- Changes in appetite and/or weight.

Social symptoms

- Avoiding contact with friends/family
- Having problems in your family/personal life
- Neglecting your hobbies/interests.

Depression ranges from being mild to severe. A diagnosis of depression is made if people have experienced four to five of these symptoms for the past two weeks. You can use the PHQ-9 questionnaire which follows to assess your mood.

There are many different options for treating depression, including medication and psychological therapy. There are very effective treatments available for depression, so it is important to seek help.

How does depression affect weight loss?

Depression can affect weight loss because eating patterns can change, especially if someone has a tendency to comfort eat when they are feeling low. In addition, depression really affects motivation so that it feels very effortful to do things. This means it can be difficult to shop and prepare the right foods. Symptoms of depression can affect activity levels, too. People may stop going out and spend more time at home or return home as soon as possible if they do have to go out.

People can often get trapped in a vicious cycle of depression, and it can feel difficult to break out of it. Depression tends to breed

Over the last 2 weeks, how often have you been bothered by any of the following problems?	Not at all	Several days	More than half the days	Nearly every day
1 Little interest or pleasure in doing things	0	1	2	3
2 Feeling down, depressed or hopeless	0	1	2	3
3 Trouble falling or staying asleep or sleeping too much	0	1	2	3
4 Feeling tired or having little energy	0	1	2	3
5 Poor appetite or overeating	0	1	2	3
6 Feeling bad about yourself – or that you are a failure or have let yourself or your family down	0	1	2	3
7 Trouble concentrating on things, such as reading the newspaper or watching television	0	1	2	3
8 Moving or speaking so slowly that other people could have noticed? Or the opposite – being so fidgety or restless that you have been moving around a lot more than usual	0	1	2	3
9 Thoughts that you would be better off dead or of hurting yourself in some way	0	1	2	3
	PHQ-9 total score			

Figure 8.3 PHQ-9 mood screening questionnaire

If you checked off any problems, how difficult have those problems made it for you to do your work, take care of things at home or get along with other people?

Not difficult at all   Somewhat difficult   Very difficult   Extremely difficult

To work out your depression score, add up the numbers you circled for questions 1 to 9. You can then see which of the categories below your score falls into.

5–9 minimal symptoms

10–14 minor depression

15–19 moderate depression

20+ severe depression

depression too – the negative thinking caused by depression continues to make people feel depressed which means that they have more negative thoughts . . . and on it goes.

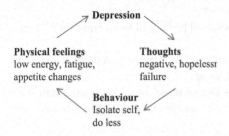

Figure 8.4 Vicious cycle of depression

Strategies to manage depression

The following sections will focus on ways of managing and changing the behaviour and thinking patterns associated with depression – this is the most helpful and effective place to start improving your mood.

Behavioural activation

When people are depressed, they often stop doing things because it can feel as though it will take too much effort or be too difficult. However, when people do less, it means they have fewer opportunities to lift their mood. Research tells us that some important features of behaviours help with depression. Engaging in activities that give you a sense of pleasure or a sense of achievement/competence is particularly helpful. Engaging in such activities stimulates the body to release natural antidepressants. It may feel as if you have to push yourself to do these things at first. It may also take some time before you start enjoying things or getting pleasure out of these activities in the way that you used to, but it is really important to keep going: it will improve.

If you think about the type of activities we do, we can split them as follows:

1) **Routine.** These are activities we do regularly. They include having a shower, cooking, shopping and taking the dog for a walk.
2) **Necessary.** These are activities that are important, and where there are consequences if we do not do them. This includes paying bills, attending appointments, taking the children to school, etc.
3) **Pleasurable.** These are activities that you previously enjoyed doing or things that you think you might enjoy doing. These obviously vary between people according to our preferences and interests. Examples may include seeing friends, going to the cinema, going for a walk and taking photos.

Have you stopped doing certain things because of your low mood? Which category do these fall into?

What things do you think it would be helpful to increase? Which category do they fall into?

Order these activities by how easy or difficult you think they would be and start with those that are easier.

Start planning to do one or two of these things each day. Start with the ones that you feel are easier to manage and then work up to the more difficult activities.

Depressed thinking habits

Depression affects the way that people think – they often start to view themselves, the world and the future negatively. It is like looking at the world through dark glasses – everything gets tinted with that negative, depressed perspective. When people are depressed, they tend to pay lots of attention to the negative thoughts they have, and this magnifies them – they dominate our minds and people tend to get "locked into" these negative thoughts.

Another feature of depression is that people tend to get stuck going over and over the same negative thoughts. These thoughts can worm their way into our minds, and it can be difficult to escape or switch off from them. This pattern of ruminative, negative thinking that dominates our thoughts makes it difficult to step back and keep things in perspective.

It is helpful if you can start to identify whether you are stuck in any thinking traps which are driving your depression and which will negatively cloud your interpretation of situations.

Depressed thinking patterns

If you can start to tune into the thoughts going through your mind when you are depressed, then you can start to recognise the type of thinking

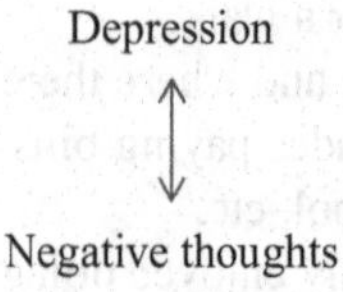

Depression

↑
↓

Negative thoughts

Figure 8.5 The reciprocal relationship between depression and negative thoughts

- **All-or-nothing thinking.** This means that you tend to think about things in extreme black or white terms, e.g. good/bad and right/wrong. There is nothing in between and no shades of grey. "I have to do things perfectly, and anything less is a failure."

- **Focusing on the negatives.** This is like having a mental filter so that only negative information gets your attention. Positive information just gets ignored or dismissed. It is like looking at the world through a pair of glasses with dark, gloomy lenses.

- **Overgeneralising.** This means being overly broad and sweeping in the conclusions we draw from events, e.g. "Everything always goes wrong" and "Nothing ever goes my way".

- **Negative self-labelling.** This is when we describe ourselves in negative and absolute terms, e.g. "I'm a complete failure".

- **Catastrophising.** This is imagining and believing that the worst possible scenario is likely to happen.

- **Mindreading.** We might assume that we know what other people are thinking – usually they focus on negative thoughts directed about us. Usually the thoughts that we assume others have about us are a reflection of our own fears or worries.

- **Should statements.** Tending to use "should" and "must" statements, usually about ourselves. These usually mean that we end up putting pressure on ourselves and set up unrealistic expectations.

Figure 8.6 Thinking habits

patterns you might have fallen into. This can be a really powerful step towards stepping back, questioning and evaluating your thoughts.

If you look at the list of thinking patterns and habits then you may well recognise a few thinking patterns and traps that you fall into. They apply to all of us to some extent!

What are your top three thinking habits when you are feeling depressed?

How to manage these thoughts

There is a well-known quote that "thoughts are thoughts, not facts". Our thoughts are our personal view of the situation, but this does not mean that they are an accurate reflection. When people are depressed or low, they get stuck in negative thinking habits, but there are alternative ways of viewing things that are likely to be more realistic and/or helpful. However, it is important to note that it is not as simple as just thinking positively about things!

Complete this diary to record any times when you notice a shift in your mood. It will help you to become more aware of the triggers and the thinking patterns that are likely to affect your emotions.

Day/time/situation	Trigger	Mood	Thought	Thinking habit	Alternative thoughts e.g. What is the evidence? How might someone else view it?

Figure 8.7 Diary to identify triggers and thoughts that affect your mood

It can be useful to write down some of the thoughts that go through your mind when you are feeling low. Just the process of writing down what you are thinking when you feel depressed can give you some perspective. Getting the thoughts out of your head and onto paper can also stop them from just going round and round in your head.

Managing the influence/power of thoughts

You can use the following questions to help you get unstuck from your thoughts and question them:

- How might someone else view this situation?
- What other ways of looking at it are there?
- What evidence supports your view of the situation? (It has to be factual evidence – not a feeling or an interpretation).
- Is this going to be important in a week, a month, six months?
- How realistic are those thoughts? What would a friend or loved one say to you?
- What would you say to a friend in a similar situation?

The questions above will help you to step back and challenge your thoughts. It is likely that you will find it difficult to generate these helpful or realistic thoughts at first, but it will get easier if you persist. You have to train your brain!

An alternative approach is to disengage from the thoughts. By this, I don't mean that you should ignore or avoid them. Instead, it is about acknowledging them as just being thoughts that will come and go. You can picture your thoughts as being like mental traffic – you can watch them go by like a pedestrian watching traffic pass by on a busy road. You can just watch them without needing to get involved.

Medication options

Antidepressants work by boosting or activating certain brain chemicals. There are different types of antidepressants, so it may take time to find the one that works best for you. Antidepressants won't make you feel happy, but they can help to lift the fog of depression so that you can use the other strategies that will lift your mood. It is important not to stop taking antidepressants suddenly and to work out a plan with your doctor for reducing or switching antidepressants.

If you are on antidepressants or other psychiatric medications, it is important to have regular reviews with the professional that prescribes these following surgery. Many people assume that because they have lost weight then their medication may need to be reduced, but actually, the opposite is often true due to the reduced absorption of medications.

There are nutritional deficiencies, including low levels of vitamin D and B12 and anaemia, which can contribute to low mood. These can be checked by your doctor or bariatric service and appropriate supplementation can be provided to address these deficiencies.

Suicide and self-harm

There is some evidence that suicide rates and self-harm are higher amongst people who have had bariatric surgery. It is still a very rare event but it would be remiss not to include information about it. A large review of the research on suicide rates after bariatric surgery found that the rates of suicide are around four times higher in the bariatric population compared to the general population (Peterhänsel et al. 2013). It seems that this tends to be more of a risk around the two- to three-year point after surgery. This is around the time when people may experience weight regain, alcohol issues and are likely to have fewer appointments with their bariatric service. If you are experiencing suicidal thoughts or feelings then it is important to seek help urgently. If you are in touch with a mental health team contact them urgently. If not and you feel unsafe, go to your local A&E or Emergency Room.

Alcohol issues

Bariatric surgery increases the risk of developing alcohol dependency issues for people who have gastric bypass surgery. A recent study followed people for seven years after bariatric surgery and found that one in five people who have gastric bypass surgery have problems with alcohol during this time (King et al. 2017). This seems to be because of increased sensitivity to alcohol: people become intoxicated quicker and will remain so for longer. The research shows that alcohol intake tends to increase between one to two years following surgery. It is important to be aware that not only those people who have previously had problems with alcohol are at risk. Approximately 60% of people who develop alcohol problems after surgery do not have a history of previous alcohol issues (King et al. 2012).

A man who had gastric bypass surgery developed problems with alcohol approximately six months following his operation. His alcohol intake escalated; he experienced blackouts and was admitted to hospital in a critical condition. He explains how the experience of drinking alcohol was different after surgery.

Alcohol had a very different effect on me after surgery. Whereas previously I would have been able to drink around six pints before getting drunk, I was now getting drunk after one or two pints. After a few weeks, alcohol was taking on a bigger and bigger role. I was now blacking out much quicker and my behaviour when drunk was completely unmanageable. The scary thing was that I didn't have a clue about what I had done. Other people were telling me I was doing things I would never have done ordinarily, falling down, getting aggressive and doing things which were always heartbreaking the morning after.

MF, 12 months post bypass

Alcohol problems can impact your weight loss and can also lead to nutritional deficiencies. Some of these deficiencies can be extremely serious – for example, thiamine deficiency if not addressed quickly can lead to permanent changes in vision, walking and memory (this is called Korsakoff syndrome) and is irreversible.

Problems with alcohol tend to escalate quickly after surgery, so it is extremely important to seek help from your bariatric service even if the amount of alcohol you are drinking seems relatively modest. You could also ask the bariatric service to liaise with your local alcohol service, as they may need information and education about the specific problems associated with alcohol problems following bariatric surgery (including the fact that much smaller amounts of alcohol intake are considered problematic).

Summary

Many psychological adjustments occur after bariatric surgery. These include changes in terms of how you now view yourself and how other people view you and relate to you. These changes can be very positive but can feel challenging and anxiety provoking at the same time. Bariatric surgery creates a window of opportunity to improve psychological health, so it's important to take full advantage of this.

References

Ivezaj, V., and Grilo, C.M. 2015. When mood worsens after gastric bypass surgery: characterization of bariatric patients with increases in depressive symptoms following surgery. *Obesity Surgery*, 25 (3), 423–429. doi:10.1007/s11695-014-1402-z

King, W.C., et al., 2012. Prevalence of alcohol use disorders, *15261*. doi:10.1001/jama.2012.6147

King, W.C., et al., 2017. Alcohol and other substance use after bariatric surgery: prospective evidence from a U.S. multicenter cohort study, *13*, 1392–1402.

Peterhänsel, C., et al., 2013. Risk of completed suicide after bariatric surgery: a systematic review. *Obesity Reviews : An Official Journal of the International Association for the Study of Obesity, 14* (5), 369–82. doi:10.1111/obr.12014

White, M.A., et al., 2015. Prognostic significance of depressive symptoms on weight loss and psychosocial outcomes following gastric bypass surgery: a prospective 24-month follow-up study, 1909–1916. doi:10.1007/s11695-015-1631-9

Chapter 9

Physical activity

Physical activity is a very important part of your weight loss and maintenance plan following bariatric surgery, yet it is one of the areas that people often struggle to incorporate into their lives. This chapter focuses on incorporating and increasing physical activity as part of your lifestyle after surgery. The reasons for incorporating physical activity are reviewed alongside the recommendations for activity. The final section focuses on strategies that are useful in aiding you to work towards increasing your physical activity levels.

Many people have struggled with activity before surgery, but after the operation, it can feel much more manageable and they notice many different benefits.

> Before surgery I was struggling to walk even a few hundred yards. It was difficult to do anything. People who say, 'just exercise more' have no understanding that you just do not have the energy to do so. You reach a downward spiral where exercise is physically too hard so any motivation to do some exercise is soon killed off. Now I feel I can exercise and do a bit more each day and I can see the change in myself mentally and physically by doing so.
>
> VS, 4 years post surgery (bypass and
> revisional surgery)

What do we mean by physical activity?

People often assume that when we talk about needing to increase and regularly incorporate activity into our lives, we mean taking up a strict exercise regime. The word exercise can bring up all sorts of memories and feelings for people . . . often fairly unpleasant ones! People often assume that this means that they need to go to the gym and embark on a very high intensity exercise session which could be painful and potentially embarrassing, too. Going to the gym may suit some people, but there are many other options that people might find more manageable and enjoyable.

Different types of activity require different levels of effort and exertion. It can be helpful to rate your exertion level on a scale from 1 to 10.

Any behaviour which requires very little energy or exertion can be classified as *sedentary behaviour*. We might think about this as a 0 or 1 on our exertion scale. Examples include sitting and watching TV. Our working lives have changed dramatically over the years so many people now have jobs which involve sitting at a desk for many hours. This type of sedentary activity will contribute to weight issues. Research tells us that it is important to think about reducing sedentary behaviour because it is associated with weight gain and other physical health difficulties. We find that as obesity increases, so does the amount of time spent being sedentary. A study found that in comparison to the general population, pre-op bariatric patients spend 35% more of their time being sedentary (Bergh et al. 2017).

There are different approaches to increasing our activity. One way of doing this is to increase our *low intensity activity* by finding small ways to increase our day-to-day activity. Any activity that increases our heart rate, makes us breathe harder and makes us feel warmer counts as activity. We might think about these activities as between 2 and 5 on our exertion scales. Examples might include slow walking, taking the stairs and completing household chores.

We can also increase our activity by engaging in physical activity of a *moderate intensity*. When completing moderate activity, most people are able to hold a conversation. We can think about this as between a 5 and 8 on our exertion scale. Examples of this might include brisk walking or cycling. Finally, we can engage in *vigorous intensity activity*. In contrast to moderate activity, saying more than a few words is very tricky during vigorous activities. We can think about this as between an 8 and 10 on our exertion scale. Examples might include running or completing a vigorous gym class.

Why is physical activity important after bariatric surgery?

Physical activity is a very important part of making bariatric surgery effective and keeping weight off. We tend to focus more attention on the eating aspects of weight management, but physical activity is vital for weight loss maintenance. There is some evidence that reducing sedentary behaviour and increasing physical activity can improve physical weight loss outcomes after bariatric surgery (Bond et al. 2011). The differences in how much physical activity people engage in directly contributes to the differences seen in weight loss outcomes. Physical activity is also important for psychological and emotional wellbeing and can help people update and improve their body image.

Does physical activity affect weight loss?

The evidence indicates that physical activity makes more of a difference to weight maintenance rather than weight loss itself. This is important information because many people having bariatric surgery worry about their ability to maintain weight loss because of their previous yo-yo dieting. The knowledge that physical activity is key to keeping weight off can be empowering. There is evidence that people who lose more weight after surgery engage in more activity. A study (Mundi et al. 2014) found that those people who lost greater than 50% of their excess weight 12 months after their bariatric surgery did 120 minutes of vigorous activity, 150 minutes of moderate activity and 233 minutes of walking per week. This was in comparison to those who had lost less than 50% of their excess weight who did 40 minutes of vigorous activity, 68 minutes of moderate activity and 188 minutes of walking.

How does physical activity help with weight loss maintenance after bariatric surgery?

Over time, the body gradually becomes used to reduced food intake and tries to return to its previous higher weight through inbuilt physiological mechanisms that start to work against our weight loss efforts. This means that the best way to create weight equilibrium and stability over time is through activity. An obesity doctor, Dr. Sharma, writes a very informative and helpful blog about obesity. He uses an analogy to describe the inbuilt physiological mechanisms which make weight maintenance challenging. He talks about losing weight as trying to walk down an escalator which is going up; that is, you are walking in the opposite direction to the way the escalator is travelling. The closer you are to the top of the escalator, the faster you have to walk to stay in the same spot. This is where activity becomes crucial. It is obviously not possible (or wise) to keep making further and further reductions to your eating in order to create this energy gap – the body will simply get used to smaller and smaller amounts of fuel and adjust accordingly. This means that physical activity is the main way that your weight can remain stable.

One issue that can trip people up is that they tend to overestimate the amount of activity they are doing after surgery and so tend not to do as much as required to maintain weight. This overestimation bias is discussed in more detail later with strategies to counteract it.

Other benefits of physical activity

Whilst physical activity is important for weight loss and weight loss maintenance, the benefits go far beyond this. They also include improved physical and mental health as well as helping with positive body image.

Physical health benefits include improvements in metabolic health, cardiorespiratory functioning, body composition/strength and energy levels.

Improved mental and emotional health includes improved confidence and self-esteem. Activity affects dopamine and serotonin; both of these are neurotransmitters, which affect our mood and thinking. Regular physical activity is a natural antidepressant and is recommended as a treatment for depression. It can also help with our ability to concentrate and help with sleep issues. Often people find that they feel calmer after exercising and more are able to put things into perspective.

> Whilst my weight has remained stubbornly static, I have dropped a clothes size and mentally I feel great. I am enjoying getting outside in all weathers and seeing the countryside and wildlife. It clears the mind of stress and worries and actually makes me more effective when working or concentrating on other things.
>
> SV, now walking 10,000+ steps per day

Improved adherence to other behaviour changes

When people put more effort into doing more activity, they are more likely to stick to the eating plan too, as they don't want to undo all the effort and hard work they have just put in.

In addition, some people describe feeling more in tune with their body through doing regular activity, and this awareness can spread to other aspects including the physical effects of certain foods and how hungry or full you feel. Physical activity can help you reconnect and tune into your body.

Facilitating improvements in body image

Physical activity can help the process of updating and improving body image following surgery because people get more perceptual and physical feedback through activity and movement. As discussed in Chapter 10, there can often be a time lag for people in recognising that they have actually lost weight, and exercise can be a really useful way of updating your body image. In addition, it is helpful to get information using your different senses (not just your eyes, which are image/appearance focused) about what the body feels like and is capable of doing. Through doing regular activity you can also get regular feedback about how your body changes and improves (appearance, strength, health etc.) over time. Activity is a great way of reconnecting with the body, too. Some people have developed a very negative view of their body after many years of trying to lose weight. Activity can be a useful way of reconnecting with the body and starting to create a different type of relationship with it (not just based on weight and image) by noticing its changing capabilities.

Increasing your physical activity after bariatric surgery

When to start increasing your activity

Following bariatric surgery, it is usually recommended that people start moving as quickly as possible rather than remaining in bed. This is partly to reduce the risk of blood clots forming. When you get home from hospital, it is recommended that you focus on walking and increase the amount and distance you cover. Bear in mind that you are still recovering from surgery and your body is adjusting to having much less fuel/food, so don't push yourself too hard. The aim is to keep active and do short, frequent walks at this stage.

Any strenuous activity or exercise should be avoided until you get clearance from your surgeon that it is ok to start this. This is usually around six weeks after the operation.

Guidelines and recommendations for activity

The most consistent physical activity guidelines from the UK and US recommend aiming for at least 150 minutes of moderate to vigorous physical activity per week. The recommendation is to aim for 30 minutes per day on five days per week. It is important to note that the activity does not have to be done in one 30-minute session; you can break it up into 10-minute episodes of activity.

One study found that physical activity levels after bariatric surgery show a slight decrease in sedentary behaviour and an increase in moderate activity in the first year after surgery, and this was maintained for the three-year period of follow-up (King et al. 2015). However, it is important to note that physical activity levels were still short of recommended guidelines. It is a very common finding, that very few people do enough activity after surgery to meet the recommended physical activity guidelines.

Getting advice based on your medical circumstances

Different people may be able to help you work out an activity plan after surgery:

- Your bariatric service
- An exercise physiologist or physiotherapist
- Your GP, who may be able to refer you to an exercise programme.

It may be worth considering having a few sessions with a personal trainer if this is financially viable when you are ready to start increasing your activity. It can help you become familiar with any equipment, get into a routine and help you feel more comfortable and confident. When choosing a personal trainer, make sure they have the appropriate qualifications and are sensitive to the needs of people with weight issues. Another positive aspect of having a personal trainer is that it can help with motivation and doing regular activity – many people find that they are less likely to cancel an appointment with someone else!

Overcoming barriers to activity

Whilst we know that physical activity is an important predictor of weight loss maintenance after surgery, it is also the area that people are least likely to incorporate into their lifestyle. Less than 20% of individuals who have had bariatric surgery meet the recommended activity guidelines (Bergh et al. 2017). There can be a combination of psychological, practical and physical barriers to activity.

Physical barriers to activity may include physical health difficulties such as pain and mobility issues. Also, people sometimes find that they feel fatigued and lacking in energy for a while after their bariatric surgery, which is partly due to the recovery process and because of their reduced food intake. Issues with excess skin can also affect how much activity someone engages in.

It is important to start with small goals and to find manageable ways of increasing your activity. These might be chair exercises, doing exercises at home using online resources, walking and so on. It is helpful to get advice from a specialist exercise physiologist, physiotherapist or exercise trainer who will be able to identify activities and exercises that are manageable and helpful for your specific circumstances. Anything that is more than what you are currently doing is a step in the right direction!

Psychological barriers to activity include thoughts such as:

- I won't be able to do it.
- I won't be able to keep up.
- It will hurt and cause me pain.
- It will be really embarrassing.
- I won't enjoy it.
- People will stare and laugh at me.

Sometimes people assume that everyone else engaging in physical activity or exercise is very slim and fit – this is not the case at all. Gyms and exercise classes are full of people of different shapes and sizes. Each individual who attends will be doing so for their own reasons (e.g. to increase their fitness, to increase their strength, to lose weight): they don't go to look at other people. Everyone will have had to attend for the first time at some point – it's natural to be apprehensive and nervous. If you are going to a class or a gym, try to familiarise yourself with the location and environment beforehand. If you are going to a class for the first time, try to go a few minutes early to explain to the instructor that it is your first time. Try to give yourself credit for being brave, stepping out of your comfort zone and doing something positive for yourself!

It is important not to put too much pressure on yourself when starting to increase your activity levels; your aim is to keep doing it rather than push yourself too hard and then stop. It takes time to learn new skills and increase your stamina; use your own starting point to track your progress rather than making comparisons with other people.

People sometimes rely on past memories and experiences of activity rather than updating these to find out what they are physically able to do after losing weight. This may mean that they still believe that that they are not capable of doing certain activities or that it will be too difficult or painful. It can be motivating to reassess yourself and find out what is now possible.

Try to think about activities that you enjoy – think outside the box about activities that you enjoy that may not necessarily be what we perceive as "exercise". Examples include dancing, window shopping and walking round a museum or gallery. Keep trying different things until you find something that you find enjoyable; different things work for different people, so it may take some time to identify what works for you.

> Previously I would avoid going to the gym because I'd feel self-conscious and think that people were laughing at me or judging me. I never used to consider the fact that some people might be thinking that it was really positive that I was going. Now I've had the surgery those worries about other people don't put me off. Once I've done the activity I feel much better in myself. I feel I've got more stamina – I can do a little bit extra each week. Also I get a sense of achievement and that stays with me. I think to myself I've spent an hour sweating and exercising so 'Do I really want that cream cake?' It's just not worth it. I say to myself that 'You don't really need it because if you have it, you'll feel bad and then you'll comfort eat'. Once you've had a good, successful day then the following day when you are thinking back, it makes you feel good and that pushes me to continue.
>
> DA, 3 years post surgery

Practical barriers can include financial pressures and time management issues.

It can be challenging to find the time to do enough activity and to prioritise it when there are competing demands in our lives. If you step back and think about the things that you are spending your time doing, are they truly important? What would happen if you didn't do them? Are you doing some things on behalf of others that they could actually do themselves? For those people who are really pressed for time, it is useful to think about splitting activity into 3×10-minute bursts – this is often far more attainable.

Financial issues are also a barrier for some people, especially if they associate physical activity with attending a gym where membership can be costly. Some activities you can do are free, for example walking, or there may be free exercise classes available in your local community. There are also many online exercise classes that are free but obviously, you have to select one that is appropriate for your circumstances.

The importance of getting objective information and accurately tracking activity

It is important to track your activity so that you get accurate information about how much you are doing. People often think that they are doing far more activity than they actually are. You can track your activity by using various gadgets including Fitbits, pedometers, minutes spent being active, etc

A study by Dale Bond and colleagues (Bond et al. 2009) followed up a group of people having surgery from pre op to six months post op and asked them to complete a questionnaire about their physical activity as well as wear an accelerometer (an objective measure of how much activity an individual does). When they assessed patients six months after their operation, the participants reported a five-fold increase in moderate/vigorous physical activity, but when this was objectively assessed, their activity had not actually increased! A more recent study of people who had gastric bypass surgery 12 months previously found that less than 20% were doing enough activity to meet these guidelines. However, when people were asked to rate how much activity they believed they were doing, 80% thought they were meeting the activity targets (Bergh et al. 2017).

Why is there a mismatch? It is possible that because people often feel physically better after surgery they assume they are doing much more than they actually are. Alternatively, maybe people attribute their weight loss to surgery and don't realise how important and crucial physical activity is for weight loss maintenance.

By keeping track of how much activity you are doing, you will also be able to see how you progress and improve over time. You can also use it to set yourself goals or track your activity as part of a group. It can also unleash a competitive spirit in some people!

> Buying a Fitbit (activity tracker) has been a brilliant tool. Not only does it motivate me to do more, it has given me a competitive edge with some colleagues and we've all ended up doing more walking because of it – everyone is a winner regardless of where we rank on the scoreboard (though I am No1, ha ha!).
>
> SV, 18 months post bypass

Set realistic goals

Setting some realistic goals for yourself can help to keep you motivated and spur you on to keep going. It's a helpful way of monitoring progress and improvement over time. Some people find it helpful to work towards an organised, sponsored activity event, for example, a charity walk or a run.

Making decisions and working out a plan

- How often are you going to engage in activity?
- Do you prefer to do your activity at the start of the day or at the end?
- Do you prefer to do your physical activity alone or with someone?
- Do you prefer to do a structured activity, e.g. exercise class, or your own activity?
- What type of activity are you going to do?

Ways of reducing sedentary behaviour and increasing activity

- Limit the amount of time spent watching TV.
- Stand up every time certain events occur, e.g. when an advert comes on TV or when you get a notification on your mobile phone.
- Stand instead of sitting where possible.
- Set an alarm on your fitness tracker to alert you when you have been sedentary.
- Use stairs rather than the elevator.
- Walk instead of using public transport or driving.
- Do household chores/tasks.
- Walk over to speak to colleagues rather than phoning or emailing them.
- Go for a walk during your lunchbreak.
- Work up to walking 10,000 steps per day.
- Find things that you enjoy – keep trying different things until you find the right thing.
- Water aerobics and swimming are often good options as they are low impact on the body.

Summary

There are different approaches and strategies that you can use to reduce sedentary behaviour and to increase your physical activity. Some people find it easier to start by reducing their sedentary behaviour before moving on to work at increasing their physical activity. Finding ways of incorporating regular physical activity into your routine is very important for long-term weight loss (and to avoid weight regain) as well as for your emotional health.

References

Bergh, I., et al., 2017. Predictors of physical activity after gastric bypass – a prospective study. *Obesity Surgery*, 17, 2050–2057. doi:10.1007/s11695-017-2593-x

Bond, D.S., et al., 2009. Pre- to postoperative physical activity changes in bariatric surgery patients: self-report vs. objective measures. *Obesity*, *18* (12), 2395–2397. doi:10.1038/oby.2010.88

Bond, D.S., et al., 2011. NIH public access. *Obesity Surgery*, *21* (6), 811–814. doi:10.1007/s11695-010-0151-x.Objective

King, W.C., et al., 2015. Objective assessment of changes in physical activity and sedentary behavior: pre- through 3 years post-bariatric surgery, *Obesity*, *23* (6), 1143–1150. doi:10.1002/oby.21106

Mundi, M.S., et al., 2014. A qualitative analysis of bariatric patients' post-surgical barriers to exercise. *Obesity Surgery*, *24* (2), 292–298. doi:10.1007/s11695-013-1088-7

Chapter 10

Body image and body confidence

This chapter focuses on changes and adjustments in body image following bariatric surgery. Some body image changes after bariatric surgery are positive, but others are more challenging (for example, coping with excess skin).

Many people seeking bariatric surgery, who have struggled with their weight for many years, have a negative relationship with their bodies and poor body image. Generally, body image improves as a result of weight loss, but it is important to proactively work at updating and improving body image during the weight loss phase as this can be a buffer against weight regain. It can also help with depression and low self-esteem (Pona et al. 2015).

What is body image?

Body image is the mental image you have of your body and your appearance. It is the picture you have in your mind's eye of your body and appearance. Body image isn't just the image you have of yourself: it is also the thoughts, evaluations and feelings that are connected with this image.

There are four different aspects of body image:

The way you see yourself (perception)

Body image is the internal mental image you have of your body and your appearance. The image we have of ourselves is sometimes wildly inaccurate and differs from how others may see you. There is generally a tendency to focus on body areas that we are self-conscious about and to assume that these are more noticeable to others than they are in reality.

The way you feel about the way you look (emotional)

People may have different emotional reactions to their bodies. These emotional reactions may range from disregard to pride to disgust and repulsion. If people have experienced negative comments about their weight previously, they may have a negative emotional relationship with their body. They may experience their body as an undesirable, unacceptable object, and this obviously affects the way they feel about it.

The thoughts, beliefs and judgements you make about your body (cognitive)

These include the judgements we make about the appearance of our body and how others may view it. For some people, these thoughts can be self-critical and cruel. This also includes our beliefs about what our bodies are capable of doing.

The way you behave because of your body image (behavioural)

When a person is dissatisfied with the way they look, they may avoid certain situations (e.g. relationships) or do certain things to make themselves feel less exposed, for example, wearing baggy clothes. If people are very unhappy about their body image and have a distorted perception of how they look, this can also drive them to restrict their eating and exercise too much.

Body image before and after bariatric surgery

The dramatic and rapid weight loss that follows bariatric surgery can create sudden shifts in body image. It is a lot for your brain to deal with in a short space of time! Most people have developed a stable image of themselves (even if it is inaccurate and/or different to how others actually see them), and so when their body changes quickly, it can be a challenge for the brain to update at the same pace.

Body image is strongly influenced by the feedback we get from the outside world. Many people seeking bariatric surgery have had upsetting and shaming experiences of people judging, ridiculing or criticising them because of their weight. This experience of being stigmatised and being judged on the basis of weight can have a devastating impact on self-esteem and body image. It can lead people to feel very self-conscious about their appearance and can cause people to avoid situations because of this. It also means that people can develop a habit of being self-critical about themselves. It is as though they develop the same prejudiced attitudes to themselves that other people may express about people with weight issues.

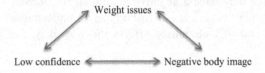

Figure 10.1 Interactions between weight, body image and confidence

This is called internalised stigma. Being overweight, negative body image and low self-confidence can become very closely entangled. Each aspect starts to affect another – so, for example, having low confidence may affect whether someone feels able to engage in exercise, or it may lead to comfort eating, which means that they continue to have weight problems and feel negatively about their body.

Indeed, wanting to improve body image can be one of the reasons why people seek surgery.

So what happens to body image after surgery? The majority of people report significant improvements in their body image and feel less concerned about their weight affecting their confidence. Generally, people feel it is less likely that they will be "picked on" or judged because of their weight. This can make them feel more comfortable and confident. People have often felt that their weight has held them back in all sorts of ways before and describe feeling that these restrictions and limitations are no longer in place.

> I feel a lot more confident now. I feel that I can approach people and not be judged on my weight. It's a massive barrier that has come down.
>
> JT, 12 months post sleeve gastrectomy

> The fact that you walk into a room and you can see people's reaction is amazing. It's such a joy. People do respond and treat you very differently.
>
> AM, 10 months post bypass

The compliments and attention that people may start to receive because of their weight loss can feel positive and motivating. The experience of receiving external feedback can feel like recognition and validation that all the hard work you are putting in is paying off. It is an external reminder that you are on the right track!

Updating your body image – the brain and body time lag after surgery

It can take time for the brain to catch up when you are going through such significant and rapid changes to your weight following surgery. The body seems to change faster than the brain. In the early stages following surgery, many people do not see themselves as being smaller or having lost weight when they look at themselves in the mirror, even though rationally they know that they have lost a large amount of weight. They often describe *knowing* that they have lost weight but *feeling* like they look the same. It can be a very confusing experience.

> At first when the weight was coming off it was so quick I couldn't keep up with it . . . I couldn't compute it. Suddenly you wake up and you realise you've got a shape and bones and there's this moment of shock. It felt quite frightening and almost like an out of body experience. I was in catch up mode and it took me ages to accept that the body I have is mine.
>
> ER, lost 76.2kg post bypass

> I didn't notice the weight loss for months and months . . . probably only a year after surgery. I just couldn't see it when I looked at photos or in the mirror. When I looked in the mirror I would still see myself as I was before surgery but I could see my clothes were getting smaller so I knew I had to be losing weight. Now it has caught up and I can notice the difference. I can see the changes in photos when I look back now.
>
> JT, lost 63.5kg in 12 months

Some people have the disconcerting experience of not recognising themselves when they look in the mirror and then realise that the image in the mirror must be them. This can sometimes be compounded when people they have not seen for a while also fail to recognise them. Many people prior to bariatric surgery have avoided mirrors, photos, buying clothes so tend not to have a very accurate or realistic perception of how they look. This means that people often don't have an accurate reference point to compare themselves to after surgery. In addition, past memories of our body image influence what we expect to see when we look in the mirror – this means that we see ourselves with our "old eyes" (not our "new eyes") rather than how we actually look now. This adds to the confusion and the short-term challenges that the brain experiences when updating and syncing your old image and your new image.

It takes time for the brain to catch up with your body, and there are some things you can do to help this. This is a way of nudging your brain into updating itself with new information about your appearance, size and image.

Strategies to update and enhance your body image

Describing what you see – not what you feel

It's important to break old patterns of avoiding mirrors and photos so that you can start to create an accurate and up-to-date image of your body and appearance. However, it's important to think about *how* you look and the content and tone of the running commentary you give. When doing this sort of exercise, it is really important to create some mental distance by stepping back from the mirror image to describe it as if you are looking at a stranger. This is because old experiences of being self-critical may taint how you perceive yourself now. It is important to create some emotional distance.

A psychologist, Thomas Cash, has written about ways of improving body image. One of the exercises he uses to help people improve their body image is described below – when you read the instructions, the exercise may sound daunting or odd, but please try it and see what happens.

Exercise

Find a full-length mirror to look in. It can sometimes help to either use a different mirror than the one you are used to using or move the mirror to a different place to where it was before. These may seem like odd suggestions, but the idea is to make things unfamiliar to minimise the chance of your "old eyes" interfering or tainting your perception of your up-to-date image.

Now describe your body as you would to a blind person who wants to know what you look like or to an artist who is trying to sketch you without seeing you. It is important to describe your body in a factual way rather than evaluate or make comments. Describe each part of your body and say it aloud. Do not use critical or exaggerating words (e.g. "bad hair", "fat bum"). When you have finished going through this description, spend a minute looking at your total reflection – focus on your body as a whole, not separate parts.

After finishing this exercise, think about what you noticed and how you felt. It's important to repeat this exercise a few times.

It may be helpful to create some distance by pretending to step into the shoes of someone else who you respect and admire, and try doing the commentary from their perspective. There are no restrictions on who you can choose: it can be anyone, including people you know and those you admire from afar. When I have previously done this exercise, people have chosen figures such as favourite relatives, close friends, Michelle Obama, Nelson Mandela, former teachers and so on. You can now ask yourself, what would they say if they were looking at your image? How would they describe your appearance? This can often be a slightly easier starting point than describing your appearance from your own perspective.

Paying equal attention to areas of your body

We are often tuned into focusing in on the parts of our appearance that we are unhappy or dissatisfied with, so we need to balance this out so that we are less biased. This means paying equal attention to areas that we are neutral about, areas we like and those we dislike.

Areas that you dislike:

Areas that you are neutral about (neither like nor dislike):

Areas that you like:

How easy was it for you to do this exercise? Often people find it much easier to generate the list of areas that they dislike, and it can be difficult for people to find areas that they like – this doesn't mean that those areas don't exist; it's just that they are not used to noticing them.

Change over time

It can be useful to use photos as another way of creating distance and updating your image. If you have a series of photos that you have taken over time, this can really help people to start noticing and spotting the differences in their shape. If you start taking photos to record your weight loss, it is helpful to take them in the same place so that you can create a stable reference point to evaluate changes – for example, some people stand in a doorway so that they can see the gaps around their silhouette change over time.

There may be other reference points you can use to update your body image, too. These include:

- trying on clothes you used to wear before surgery;
- trying old belts on and seeing the change in which hole you use;
- checking how rings fit on your fingers;
- seeing if you can feel collarbones, ankles or hips.

Updating and reminding yourself about how your body functions now

People usually find that it is much easier to physically do things after weight loss, and it is important to pay attention to these changes, rather than just focusing on the weighing scales and appearance changes. It is helpful to broaden out your perception of what the body can do now that you have lost weight. This involves gathering information about what you are able to do now that might not have been possible or as easy before. This can help you to reconnect with your smaller body. This is a huge mental shift from before surgery when people are often focused on what is *not* possible.

Examples include:

- being able to choose clothes that you actually like
- being more able to physically do things and be more active
- being more able to do things that you enjoy without worrying about your weight, e.g. fasten seatbelts, go on rollercoasters etc.
- being more able to be an active parent
- being less dependent on others to do things for you.

Exercise and movement are important ways to reconnect with the body and to start to create a different relationship with it. It helps to update your perception of what the body can do and what an amazing, adaptable resource it is. Exercise and movement also help you to use different senses (not just your eyes) to help you to collect more information about your body.

Updating your behaviour

Part of updating your perception of what your body can now do is making sure that you are no longer using some of the adaptations or avoidant behaviours you might have used before because of your size. These include things like standing up on public transport because of fear that you may not fit in the seats, walking around (rather than through) obstacles in shops for fear that you may not fit through, avoiding travelling for fear that airplane seatbelts may not fit and so on. If these behaviours continue then it maintains the idea that your size hasn't changed and that you are still too large to navigate these things. By approaching and testing out these situations, you can get evidence to update and challenge those old beliefs.

Shopping and clothes

There are many positive aspects of being able to buy smaller clothes, including having a greater choice of clothes available rather than being limited to clothes stocked by shops that solely cater for larger people. This can also be an important way to update your body image – for example, knowing that your clothes sizes have reduced significantly can be an important bit of evidence to nudge your brain into recognising that you have lost weight. Some people avoid going shopping because of concerns about their body image, but this is likely to perpetuate the problem of inaccurate body perception because they don't have any accurate information to work with.

Choosing clothes and shopping for clothes can be a learning process requiring the development of new skills. For example:

- learning how to shop and what suits you due to increased choice
- learning how fitted clothes feel on your body
- learning how to manage excess skin when making choices about clothes
- learning what size you are in which particular shop.

Many people have wardrobes that are full of clothes they have grown both into, and out of, on numerous occasions, so it is difficult to truly believe that the same won't happen again. It is important to get rid of old clothes – by keeping them, it's like having an insurance policy in case of weight regain. Keeping these clothes is a reflection of low confidence and self-belief in your ability to maintain your weight. This can become a self-fulfilling prophecy.

Getting feedback from others

Another way to update your body image is to ask others for feedback on the changes and differences that they can see. This can sometimes be an easier place to start than trying to spot the differences ourselves. They have a slightly different perspective as a witness to your weight loss, so it is easier for them to give feedback. Obviously you have to think carefully about who you ask and what you want them to comment on.

Updating your perception of size in comparison with others

Some people describe always having been "the biggest person in the room", and because this belief has become so firmly entrenched over the years it doesn't change, despite weight loss. This is particularly likely for people who have felt embarrassed and self-conscious about their weight. These old memories and fears get in the way of updating their body image. This happened with a woman that was two years post surgery who was anxious about an upcoming Christmas party and was convinced she was still "the largest person in the room". She believed 100% that others would view her this way and stare at her. She was previously a size 24 and was now a clothes size 14. She estimated the dress sizes of the other people in the group of friends she would be attending the party with – in reality, she was actually the smallest size! Again, the important principles are to step back and look at the evidence behind the beliefs – are these still accurate beliefs or do they need updating?

Coping with feelings of visibility

Some people struggle with feeling more visible and noticeable to other people as a result of losing weight. This is more likely to be an issue for those people who have experienced abusive experiences in the past (e.g. sexual abuse). They sometimes feel frightened that as they become smaller, they will attract more attention and predatory behaviour.

> Part of the comfort eating was to have a fat blanket around me that hid me because I didn't want to look sexually attractive. I didn't want people to look at me and the weight stopped that. And then as the weight started dropping off I became more anxious about the attention I would attract – that was pretty scary and something I

didn't want. If I saw someone looking at me I would just want to scream at them 'F*** off, looking at me'. It took me a while to get out of baggy clothes that hid me to wearing more fitted clothes. Even now I feel a bit uncomfortable if someone looks at me.

ER, 15 months post bypass

This usually passes and gets easier over time – again, the brain just needs time to catch up. It is helpful to question your thinking and the likelihood of any predictions you are making in the here and now. This is part of a process of updating old fears and reassessing them in your current situation.

Seeking support

The experience of massive weight loss after bariatric surgery and all the other adjustments and issues that arise because of this are unique. This is where support groups can be very helpful. Your bariatric service may also offer a buddy system so you can be paired up with someone else who is going through the same process.

Distress and coping with excess skin

One of the biggest challenges that people experience following bariatric surgery is coping with the excess or loose skin that they are likely to experience following massive weight loss. Over 70% of people develop excess skin after bariatric surgery (Baillot et al. 2013). One study found that 75% of women and 68% of men wanted body-contouring surgery to remove this excess skin (Kitzinger et al. 2012). Areas of particular concern, in order, are the stomach/abdomen, breasts and thighs. Excess skin can have physical effects and affect physical functioning. It can cause problems with rashes, infections, ulceration, personal hygiene and mobility. It can also make it difficult to exercise. It can make it difficult to have sexual relationships or be intimate with others.

Most people are aware that they are likely to have excess skin after bariatric surgery (bariatric surgery services should raise this as a potential issue before surgery). However, even though this discussion has taken place it can be difficult for people to truly picture or imagine what it might be like to experience excess skin and it can therefore be a shock.

People vary in their reactions to excess skin. Some people describe their excess skin as being something that they feel proud of because it is a reminder of how much weight they have lost, that is, if they hadn't made a success of bariatric surgery then they wouldn't have excess skin.

In this way, they view it as a battle scar to be proud of. For others, the appearance and feel of excess skin can create strong emotional reactions, and they describe feelings of disgust and repulsion.

> My excess skin is really difficult to cope with. When I look in the mirror, I just think I look like a balloon that has been popped with wrinkly, loose skin everywhere.
>
> AG, 3 years post bypass

It can be very upsetting to have to adjust to feeling physically different or "abnormal" after bariatric surgery. Excess skin can also act as a reminder about previous weight problems, and some people worry that whilst the skin is still there they could regain weight and "grow back" into it. Others tend to misinterpret their excess skin as meaning they are still overweight.

> I have got loads of excess skin and it makes me feel that I haven't really lost weight. Although it might not be fat, it still looks like fat and it's a constant reminder every day.
>
> VH, 18 months post bypass

Some people may blame themselves for the excess skin and view it as a punishment for not having lost weight earlier in their lives. Whereas prior to surgery, excess weight was the main source of distress for people, the attention can shift to excess skin. Now that weight is less of a pressing issue, the focus and priorities can shift.

In the next section, we will review different options including psychological ways of coping and living with excess skin. Information is also provided about accessing body-contouring surgery and non-surgical options to manage excess skin.

Coping with excess skin

It would be misleading to pretend that psychological strategies are going to completely eradicate any distress about excess skin. The aim of these strategies is to help you find ways of coping that make it possible to live with excess skin.

Managing self-attacking thoughts

The type of thoughts that people may experience about their excess skin is often very self-critical and self-attacking. These thoughts can be very distressing. They can be such a harsh and punishing way to relate to your body. Would you speak to anyone else in the same way about their body?

It can be helpful to start developing a sense of compassion for the body. Your body is the container of your history, of your experiences, and it will carry you into the future. Developing compassion for the body involves being thankful for the functions that it undertakes, what it does for you and what it enables you to do. Your body is a vessel of your history, your experiences and your personality.

Respect for what the body does

It is easy to become preoccupied with the body, particularly for those people who are unhappy or disappointed with the appearance of their body after bariatric surgery. Before surgery, it is very difficult for people to truly picture or imagine what their bodies may look like after weight loss and how any excess skin may look. Sometimes people have to readjust their expectations and hopes about how their body may look after surgery. The focus can sometimes shift from being distressed and upset about being overweight to being distressed about excess skin. This focus on body image and appearance means that people may not pay much attention to what their bodies can do now that they have lost weight. This isn't about glossing over how distressing excess skin can be: it is about trying to cope and remember some of the positive aspects of losing weight.

The aim is to try to balance your thinking so that you don't just focus all your attention on the negative aspects of weight loss.

> If you rewind and remember your original reasons for losing weight and your goals, what were they?
>
> Have you reached or achieved these?
>
> What can you physically do now that you were unable to do before? E.g. stamina, flexibility, strength.

Although the excess skin is problematic and distressing, it may be that on balance, your overall situation is still better than before surgery. It is very rare for people to wish that they hadn't had the surgery done even though there are still problems and challenges to cope with.

Looking at the whole rather than zooming in

There is a tendency for people to zoom in and focus on the areas of their body that they are concerned about – for example, focusing on the excess skin on their arms or thighs. This sometimes means people touch and manipulate their skin in these areas. This just reinforces the focus and distress caused by it. We can get a distorted perception by spending a lot of time magnifying just one area because that is our area of concern. As mentioned previously, it helps to broaden out your body image perception and identify areas you dislike, like and feel neutral about.

Self-consciousness about excess skin

People sometimes assume that the body areas that they are self-conscious about are highly visible to others and that others will pay the same amount of attention to them. If you step back and think about it, how often do you just focus on one or two areas of someone's body? What is most noticeable to you about someone's appearance? For most people, it is their smile or their eyes.

Making a distinction between excess skin and "fat"

Sometimes people assume that the excess skin that they have is weight that they still have to lose rather than accepting that it is excess skin – this appears to be more of an issue for people with excess skin around their abdomen/stomach. It is important to make the distinction between excess skin and "fat", as otherwise people can feel that they have failed to lose enough weight and go on a more radical, restrictive diet which is unhealthy.

Tackling avoidance

People sometimes start to avoid situations because of their concerns about their excess skin. Avoidance is a coping strategy for managing anxiety. Whilst it might make people feel less anxious in the short term, it means that their choices and decisions become restricted because they are convinced that something awful would happen if they faced the situation. Anxiety can start to rule your decision-making.

Avoidance also keeps alive the person's beliefs that there is something "wrong" with their body that needs to be concealed from others. It means that they never get to find out that others don't share those beliefs or even notice the area they are concerned about.

Are there things that you are avoiding because of your excess skin (or how you feel about your body)?

What is the effect of this avoidance? What does it stop you doing?

When people start to do things that they have previously avoided, it is likely to feel anxiety provoking at first. The more you do it, the easier it will become. The only way to find out that the worst case scenario is unlikely to happen is to approach the situation. Even if the worst case scenario were to happen, people generally find out that it is nowhere near as bad as they predicted.

Impact of excess skin on new or existing relationships

The prospect of starting a new relationship can be both exciting and challenging at the same time! It can be difficult for people to decide if they want to tell potential partners about their previous weight and weight loss. Depending on their specific circumstances, they may also need to work out when and what to say about any excess skin too.

Some people may have previously avoided relationships because of embarrassment about their weight and may start to attract more romantic attention as they lose weight. Some people still feel that it is "safer" to avoid relationships because of difficulties in explaining their excess skin to partners or for fear they will be rejected because of it. If people avoid relationships as a way of avoiding potential shame or rejection, their confidence is likely to remain low. It keeps alive the possibility of shame and rejection whilst in reality this may not actually happen. It is like having an insurance policy that you might not need. Of course, it obviously isn't possible to guarantee that people won't be insensitive or hurtful: that is a possibility in any relationship.

Everybody has areas of their body that they are less happy about or even embarrassed about – it's a pretty universal phenomenon. In addition, there is always a difference between our clothed appearance and what we actually look like naked – having excess skin can heighten this contrast and worry about how a partner may react. Again, it is important to remember that you are likely to be far more aware of it than your partner is. Also, they are probably focused on areas of their own body that they are concerned or self-conscious about!

There is more information about relationship issues in Chapter 11.

Accessing body-contouring surgery

It can be challenging to access body-contouring surgery unless privately funded. The funding guidelines are likely to vary from area to area, so it is important to find out about these.

It is important to consider the impact of having surgery on one area on how you will feel about the remaining areas. Sometimes the focus of distress then moves on to another area. Also, there may be a marked contrast between the area where you have had surgery and the areas where you still have excess skin.

Most services recommend waiting until you have been weight stable for a decent period of time after bariatric surgery before considering body-contouring surgery. For most people, this is at least two years after their bariatric operation. The reason is that if someone has body contouring too soon and they continue to lose weight, they are likely to experience more excess skin. Most plastic surgeons recommend that if you are having multiple surgeries then these should be done in different stages rather than all at once.

If you want to find out more about body-contouring surgery then speak to your bariatric team. It is also important to do plenty of research and to have realistic expectations. If you are considering private body-contouring surgery, check the credentials of the surgeon and that they are registered with a regulatory board.

Non-surgical options

Body-contouring surgery is not necessarily an option for everyone. This may be because of financial restrictions, not wanting to have further surgery or just preferring to live with excess skin. Some non-surgical options are outlined below.

Exercise. Exercise will improve your health and body image, and it's a very important part of long-term weight maintenance. However, it is important to be honest about the fact that it will not get rid of excess skin. It will not revert your skin to how tight or firm it was before you developed weight problems. Skin only has a certain amount of elasticity, and once it has stretched beyond a certain point for a prolonged period, it is not possible for it to snap back.

Skin problems. Some people develop skin irritations, chafing and odour in their skin folds. Speak to your doctor or bariatric service, and they will be able to recommend creams and treatments that will help you to manage it.

Support underwear. There are lots of different types of support and compression underwear available, and people often find this helpful in managing and holding in their excess skin.

Summary

There are a range of body image issues that can arise as a result of weight loss after bariatric surgery – many of these are positive adjustments, but there are also challenges to negotiate. It takes time for the brain to update – the body changes faster than the brain! This is why it is so important to proactively work at updating your body image following weight loss and to use strategies to improve how you feel about your body – not just its appearance, but also the way it functions and what it is now capable of doing.

References

Baillot, A., et al., 2013. Impact of excess skin from massive weight loss on the practice of physical activity in women. *Obesity Surgery*, 23 (11), 1826–1834.

Cash, T. F., 2008. *The body image workbook: an eight step program for learning to like your looks*. Oakland, CA: New Harbinger Publications.

Kitzinger, H.B., et al., 2012. After massive weight loss: patients' expectations of body contouring surgery. *Obesity Surgery*, 22 (4), 544–548.

Pona, A.A. et al., 2015. Psychological predictors of body image concerns 3 months after bariatric surgery. *Surgery for obesity and related diseases: official journal of the American Society for Bariatric Surgery*, 12(1), pp.188–193.

Chapter 11

Changes in relationships

Weight loss after surgery can lead to changes in intimate, romantic relationships as well as our relationships with family and friends. The decision to have bariatric surgery is usually made by an individual, but it clearly has an impact on other people in our lives. This network of people can react in ways that either help or hinder with the changes that arise after surgery. The differences in the level of support available will affect how easily someone adjusts and maintains changes to eating and activity levels after surgery.

People sometimes feel uncomfortable about putting their needs first when making the decision to have bariatric surgery because they know it will impact on others. This impact can be positive, but it can also create issues and ripples within relationships. What do those around you think about your decision to have bariatric surgery? Are they willing to help, support and, if necessary, change alongside you? If not, are you prepared to make the changes despite the potential distractions or lack of active support?

Family and social relationships

The level of support someone has can have a really important effect on whether they adopt or drop health behaviours that either help or prevent weight loss maintenance (Pratt et al. 2016). It is important to consider what impact food has played in your relationships with partners, family and friends. For many people, eating has become a central aspect of spending time together – it is like the glue that connects people. In fact, we are socialised into behaving this way. We are encouraged to use food to celebrate, for example, at birthdays, Christmas, leaving parties and so on. However, after surgery it is unlikely that you will be able to connect through food in the same way, and this can affect your sense of connection and intimacy with others and vice versa. Furthermore, if you are losing weight and others around you are staying the same (or putting on weight), this creates some changes in relationships, too. It is helpful to talk about these things before surgery in order to prepare for the changes ahead and how these will be managed within your relationship. This is obviously a greater challenge for those people who prefer not to disclose they are having/have had bariatric surgery.

Reappraising your friendships

Many people who have had bariatric surgery describe how some of their friendships changed after they lost weight, and that they have even lost friendships. One reason for this is that sometimes, people start to question the friendship choices they have previously made and whether they have "settled" for friendships that are unsatisfactory and unfulfilling.

Weight loss can also be a threat to the status quo of friendships and a person's position within those groups. For example, when someone loses weight, they may no longer be the largest person in the group (the "big friend"). Or weight loss may mean that they become an outsider as they no longer "fit in" with the group. Sometimes friends can become jealous or envious of weight loss and distance themselves because of this or become competitive about losing weight. Friends may try to sabotage weight loss efforts by encouraging people to engage in "old" behaviours in an attempt to maintain the status quo. Friends can also be vocal about their views on bariatric surgery, with some viewing it as a "quick fix" or a "cheat" and therefore appearing to dismiss the effort and changes that people are making alongside the surgery. Obviously, these challenges and ruptures are not inevitable, and friends can be a huge source of support and encouragement.

It may be useful to think about how you will manage social situations with friends. A study by some researchers (Romo 2017) found that people use a range of strategies to "fit in" with friends and their social group, and this sometimes involves concealing or modifying their weight loss strategies. Some of the strategies described include accepting food and then disposing of it, having small amounts of unhealthy food given to them, designating "cheat" days and avoiding social situations. One study found that if people are very clear and vocal about their health-related reasons for continuing with their weight loss approach, then this seems to be less threatening and more acceptable to others (Romo 2017). This is likely to lead to fewer attempts to lead you astray or persuade you to do things that aren't compatible with your goals.

Strategies

- If possible, prepare people beforehand by letting them know about what you are doing, your reasons and what may be different. This may also include letting them know about how those changes may affect the way you socialise or spend time together.
- Set ground rules for yourself and decide how much you are prepared to compromise and modify your eating to "fit in".
- Reassure people that this is a decision and choice you have made and that you are not judging them for their choices and decisions.
- Suggest different shared activities other than eating.

Romantic relationships

There is often a blend of positive shifts as well as challenges to negotiate within romantic relationships after bariatric surgery. It is inevitable that there will be some relationship changes but these can present positive opportunities; it is not necessarily a negative thing. It is a myth that there are very high rates of divorce after bariatric surgery – the evidence demonstrates that those who have healthy relationships before surgery continue to do so after surgery. However, losing weight can worsen or destabilise relationships that were problematic or less healthy to begin with.

Changes after surgery can affect the status quo of relationships and this can be unsettling. For some couples, being overweight and sharing certain eating behaviours may have been an important bond in the relationship. If someone has bariatric surgery and loses a significant amount of weight and their partner remains overweight, then this can also present some challenges and changes to the relationship. Obviously, these challenges are not inevitable. They differ for individuals and they can be worked through if you are aware of them (and your partner is receptive to working on these changes, too).

Positive changes in existing romantic relationships

Some of the positive changes in relationships include:

- **Improved health and increased energy.** This means being more able to do things together that may have previously not been possible. There is a sense of feeling less inhibited and restricted by weight-related issues.
- **Increased confidence and mood.** This is linked to being more able to try new things and/or engage in activities.

- **Reduced dependency on partner.** As people lose weight, they may regain a greater sense of independence, and this means they may be less dependent on their partner to do things for them, e.g. personal care and household tasks. However, this can involve a loss of a "caring" role for their partner and means that the roles in the relationship need to be redefined.
- **Increased sociability.** As confidence improves following weight loss, people generally start to become more outward-looking. They feel less need to hide away. These reduced feelings of stigmatisation make it easier and more possible to interact with others.
- **Working together on eating changes and activity changes.** This can be a shared venture.
- **Increased sense of intimacy and closeness.** This could be increased attraction and a rediscovery of relationship.
- **Increase in sexual interest and desire.** There is an increase in sexual activity and enjoyment by people who had bariatric surgery 12 months ago (Camps, et al. 1996).

Possible challenges

Partner's role and attitude to change

The person choosing to have surgery is prepared to make changes and is ready to embrace all the opportunities that weight loss can bring to them. However, this doesn't necessarily mean that partners will feel the same way. A recent study (Wallwork et al. 2017) interviewed the partners of people who'd had bariatric surgery and described them as ranging from being "bystanders" to working "hand in hand" with their partner. One study (Kluever Romo et al. 2014) looking at the effect of bariatric surgery on relationships, found differences between partners who sought to maintain the status quo in relationships versus those that embraced change. Sometimes, partners want things to remain the same, and this means that they can resist changes. For example, they may bring tempting foods into the house and eat them in front of you. It is important to remember that your partner did not opt to have surgery and all the changes connected to it. Obviously, it is helpful if partners make changes with you, but it's not necessarily guaranteed. This is likely to be something you need to discuss and negotiate.

There are different factors that can affect how partners may feel about the changes connected with bariatric surgery. These include whether they have weight issues themselves and the extent to which food and eating was a shared activity or a bonding activity before.

We used to comfort eat together and that was a bond for us. Now it is difficult to work out how we connect. It has exposed that gap in our relationship. It makes you question when do we actually connect now? You have to put in different things to keep that partner relationship going now that food and weight aren't things we have in common.

ER, 15 months post bypass

For the individual having bariatric surgery, they are usually making an active decision to improve and change their life, and this often opens up different possibilities and opportunities for them. However, the partner who has not had bariatric surgery may remain in the same situation (whether this is because of their weight or other factors), and this can create a sense of distance. For some people, it can start to feel as though they are starting to move in a different direction from their partner.

Sabotage attempts

Sabotage attempts may be intentional or unintentional. This means that you need to stay vigilant to others sending you astray. It's important to realise that these sabotage attempts aren't usually for malicious or hostile reasons. Non-weight-loss partners may attempt to pull their partners back to the previous goal (i.e. a less healthy lifestyle) to re-establish the stability in the relationship.

Examples of sabotage attempts include repeatedly offering inappropriate foods, buying food gifts for you, cooking inappropriate foods, serving large portions and encouraging you to eat more. There are different strategies that you may need to use, including eating separate meals in order to ensure you are having "bariatric appropriate" meals. Ask partners to keep any tempting treat foods separate (e.g. they may keep them in the car or have their own cupboard). You may have to consider giving away or leaving food that partners may have bought you as a treat − if you eat it then you will encourage them to keep buying it for you. Let your partner know about other ways they can treat you that don't involve buying inappropriate foods, for example, buying you flowers, music you like and so on.

Increased awareness/criticism of partner's weight and eating behaviour

Some people who have had surgery find that they become far more aware of their partner's eating and weight as they lose weight. They can start to view their partner's eating differently as their perspective changes on what is "normal" eating. This means they can see their partner's eating through different eyes and become critical or even disgusted by their eating behaviour (and possibly irritated at their lack of change). This can have wider repercussions in the relationship as the power dynamics shift. For the person who has had bariatric surgery, their partner's continuation of old eating habits can serve as a difficult reminder of the past, thereby triggering a disgust or rejection reaction.

> The weight loss is so quick and it drives you. It's easy to forget that other people haven't had the "magic opportunity" I had which meant that I no longer wanted to eat in the same way. I didn't want to comfort eat anymore. It dramatically changed my outlook on everything. I got very frustrated and angry with my husband for not changing and I had to keep reminding myself that his journey will be longer than mine. It is very hard for him to change. I think it's made him feel worse as he's not been able to keep up with those changes . . . it's hard to talk about it in our relationship and it causes some pressure and tension. We are at different stages in our life and time is moving on.
>
> RE, 13 months post sleeve gastrectomy

> I started seeing my husband in a different way after I lost weight – I'd look at how much food he was eating and I felt disgusted by it even though it hadn't changed since my surgery. I started noticing how little care and attention he was paying to himself . . . he was starting to get a beer belly and he wasn't doing anything about it. He would just sit there on the sofa and carry on eating in the same way.
>
> AE, 18 months post bypass

It is important to remember that it is *your* weight and eating behaviour that has changed through bariatric surgery – you are in a different position now, and you are likely to be seeing things differently. You could try asking your partner if their weight or eating is something they are concerned about or want to change – if it is, then you have got some scope to offer help, but if they do not want to make changes then you will need to accept this and focus on your own changes.

Changes in opportunities

One of the benefits of losing weight after surgery is that things feel more possible and manageable, which means that the future feels more hopeful with opportunities. However, this may not be the same for your partner. It can feel uncomfortable and even guilt inducing for the person who has lost weight after surgery. This quote below is from a man who found that his life improved after bariatric surgery, yet his wife's situation did not:

> Losing weight meant I could do many more things and I started to think about my future differently. I felt that things were getting much better for me but staying the same or even getting worse for my wife and I felt really guilty about that. A few times she made comments about how she was getting left behind.
>
> HW, 20 months post bypass

The improvements in confidence that often happen after surgery may mean that people become more assertive in expressing their needs or wants. This can affect partners who may have been used to making the decisions or taking a lead in things. This shift in the power dynamics leads to a further adjustment in terms of how relationships will work in future. Again, this can be a positive as well as a negative. It is important to keep communicating about these issues.

Partner insecurity

Sometimes weight loss and the subsequent shifts in self-esteem and confidence can leave a partner feeling insecure and worrying that their partner will now leave them. Partners may be concerned and worried that because their partner has lost weight, they will no longer want to remain in a relationship with them. Again, it's an example of a potential threat to the status quo.

It is obviously important to communicate about these issues and to talk about changes. It is important to spend time together and to engage in shared activities – this can help to reassure partners that you want to spend time with them. This also involves not letting weight and eating become the defining issue in a relationship and making space for other things.

Try to involve your partner in the weight loss process if possible. They may feel like they are not part of the process or experience and therefore try to exert some sort of control. Research shows that it's helpful for couples to view weight management as a shared project and as something that they work on together as a team (Ferriby et al. 2015). This means negotiating healthy changes together if possible.

At the same time as hoping that your partner will be supportive and work as a team with you, it's also important to be realistic that you can't necessarily expect that they will sign up to adopt the post-op bariatric eating plan. This is why it is important to have transparent conversations about the impact of changes and how you will negotiate and manage these in your relationship.

Sexual functioning

Before bariatric surgery, many people have experienced difficulties with physical intimacy including problems with sexual functioning, low libido and avoidance of sexual encounters (Goitein et al. 2015). These difficulties with sexual functioning are related to a combination of physical and psychological factors. About 50% of women are dissatisfied with their sexual life before surgery (Steffen et al. 2017). The evidence shows that sexual functioning improves after bariatric surgery and that people have more frequent sex and enjoy it more. After surgery, people reported getting more pleasure from sex, feeling more attractive and being less likely to get undressed in the dark (Camps et al. 1996).

The way that someone feels about their body image is a very important factor in how someone feels about sex and their enjoyment of it. The way that we perceive, evaluate and think about our bodies seems to have more of an impact on our sexual behaviour than does our actual weight or body size. Most people's body image improves as they lose weight, but it is important to proactively work at improving body image through using some of the strategies outlined previously (see Chapter 10)

Sometimes people may have had limited or reduced sexual contact with their partner before surgery, and it can feel awkward to start to re-engage in this. There are specific techniques that can help with reintroducing sexual contact into relationships – the main one is called sensate-focused exercises. Using this approach, people start to relearn about each other's bodies through touch, but this is done in a graded way. To begin with there are clear boundaries about what the limits are, and there is agreement that there is no expectation that the massage will progress to sex. This means that you may start by giving each other a back massage and over time move onto other parts of the body involving genital contact. There are different stages you can go through, and there is detailed guidance available online.

Life is often busy and there can be many competing demands for our time. We often forget or don't prioritise spending time with our romantic partner. It is important to do this as it's a way of committing and investing in the relationship. The less time you spend together, the more distant and avoidant of intimacy people tend to become. You could try setting up a regular date night. It doesn't have to be an expensive or grand occasion – it could be going for a walk together or any situation where the two of you get to reconnect.

Contemplating new relationships

Following weight loss, some people may feel that they are more interested in having relationships and are more prepared to explore this. There is some evidence that people (particularly men) avoid relationships before (Pratt et al. 2016). This can happen for various reasons including avoidance of situations where they are likely to meet potential partners, fear of rejection, shame about their body, worries about sexual functioning and so on. This means that when it comes to contemplating starting a relationship, people may feel apprehensive or be unsure about how to meet others and how to behave. This is completely natural and understandable. A good starting point is to build up your confidence by being more sociable. You can practice this by being a bit braver and speaking to people who you see frequently but don't usually speak to – for example, saying hello to someone you regularly see at the bus stop can soon progress into a conversation!

Ways of meeting potential partners:

- Through friends
- Through work
- Joining an evening class or starting a hobby
- Through voluntary work
- At a gym
- Through online dating sites or speed dating.

The key thing is to take your time getting to know your potential partner.

There are some specific issues that you may also need to consider, which include:

- **making a decision about whether you are going to let potential or new partners know about your previous weight history.** Again, there are likely to be different reactions to your previous weight and the fact that you have had bariatric surgery, so you will need to be prepared for these. Hopefully, you will have got to know the person well enough to judge whether they are likely to make supportive or upsetting comments.

• **worries about excess skin.** As relationships develop and are becoming more intimate, people sometimes have concerns about how their partner may react to seeing their excess skin. People will have different ways of dealing with this. It is important to remember that everybody will have some areas of their body that they are self-conscious about. Your potential partner is more likely to be focused on areas of their body they are concerned about rather than evaluating you! Some prefer to be completely straightforward and just explain their surgery and the effects of weight loss on their body, but this is an individual choice.

Summary

It is inevitable that bariatric surgery and its consequences will have an impact on intimate relationships, family relationships and friendships. Some of these changes may be positive, but it is likely that there will also be challenges to negotiate too. These challenges are often not anticipated and can therefore feel very disappointing and upsetting. It is an opportunity to reappraise who is in your life and whether they support or treat you in a way that you are comfortable with.

References

Camps, M., et al., 1996. Impact of bariatric surgery on body image perception and sexuality in morbidly obese patients and their partners. *Obesity Surgery*, 6 (4), 356–360. doi:10.1381/096089296765556700

Ferriby, M., et al., 2015. Marriage and weight loss surgery: a narrative review of patient and spousal outcomes. *Obesity Surgery*, 25 (12), 2436–2442. doi:10.1007/s11695-015-1893-2

Goitein, D., et al., 2015. Bariatric surgery improves sexual function in obese patients. *The Israel Medicine Journal Association*, 17 (October).

Kluever Romo, L., and Dailey, R.M., 2014. Weighty dynamics: exploring couples' perceptions of post-weight-loss interaction. *Health Communication*, 29 (2), 193–204. doi:10.1080/10410236.2012.736467

Pratt, K.J., et al., 2016. Bariatric surgery candidates' peer and romantic relationships and associations with health behaviors. *Obesity Surgery*, 26 (11), 2764–2771. doi:10.1007/s11695-016-2196-y

Romo, L.K., 2017. An examination of how people who have lost weight communicatively negotiate interpersonal challenges to weight management. *Health Communication*, 236 (February), 1–9. doi:10.1080/10410236.2016. 1278497

Steffen, K.J., et al., 2017. Sexual functioning of men and women with severe obesity before bariatric surgery. *Surgery for Obesity and Related Diseases*, 13 (2), 334–343. doi:10.1016/j.soard.2016.09.022

Wallwork, A., et al., 2017. Exploring partners' experiences in living with patients who undergo bariatric surgery. *Obesity Surgery*, 27, 1973–1981. doi:10.1007/s11695-017-2594-9

Unmet weight loss expectations and weight regain after bariatric surgery

This chapter focuses on issues that arise for people who haven't lost as much weight as they expected or have regained weight after surgery. It provides information on the rates of weight regain and poor weight loss after bariatric surgery alongside the types of behaviours associated with these patterns. The chapter includes information on strategies that people can use to help them make sense of and address suboptimal weight loss or weight regain after surgery.

People seeking bariatric surgery feel hopeful and optimistic about the difference it will make to their lives. Understandably, it can therefore be difficult for people, and indeed, for professionals, to talk about the possibility of unmet weight loss expectations and weight regain. It can be challenging for people to process information that they don't want to believe. Most people want to believe that their weight loss experience will be different after surgery, and that it will not be possible for them to regain weight. It can also be challenging to talk about these issues after surgery as people sometimes feel ashamed and that they have "failed". However, it is important to be transparent about the possibility of these problems because if you are aware of them, then you can start to tackle them.

It is also important to distinguish between the normal upward drift in weight that most people will experience over time (whether they have had bariatric surgery or not) and weight regain which is unusual. The evidence shows that most people will experience slight weight regain after bariatric surgery, usually around the two- to three-year point. One study with a follow-up period of five years reported an average weight regain of 8kg in the two- to five-year period following surgery (Aftab et al. 2014). It is not clear why this happens – it may be a combination of factors, including the normal upward drift in weight that most people experience over time plus reduced physiological feedback from the surgery alongside changes in behaviour. What we do know is that this weight increase is much less than the weight that people would have gained or regained if they had not had bariatric surgery.

The psychological effects of poor weight loss or regain can be very challenging for people to cope with. We know that psychological well-being after surgery is very closely tied in with weight loss, so that if weight loss stops or people regain some weight then this is a risk factor for poor emotional health. The experience of unmet weight loss expectations can reactivate previous beliefs about not having enough "will-power" and being a "failure". It can also trigger a dieting mindset so that people start to panic about their weight and then make radical changes (e.g. going on a "fad diet") that are not sustainable. The important thing to remember is that if you truly allow yourself to step back, assess what is happening and start to make changes, it is possible to start to lose weight again. It is never too late.

What is classified as suboptimal weight loss and weight regain?

Poor weight loss is generally defined as losing less than 50% of your excess weight loss. Weight regain is usually defined as putting on 15% (or more) of the weight you had previously lost. Recent data and evidence suggests that about 20–30% of individuals have either insufficient weight loss or excessive weight regain (Sheets et al. 2014).

How many people lose less than expected weight?

A recent study (De Hollanda et al. 2014) that looked at weight loss after bariatric surgery over an average of four years found three patterns of weight loss emerged. They defined expected weight loss as >50% of their EWL.

1)   76% of people lost weight in the expected way.
2)   5% didn't lose as much weight as expected.
3)   19% lost weight and then regained some weight.

At what point do people start to split into different weight loss groups?

The physiological effects of bariatric surgery (related to gut hormones and appetite control) tend to be very strong for the first year when most weight is lost. However, these effects tend to wear off over time, and the maintenance of weight loss becomes increasingly dependent on lifestyle and behaviour modification. Differences in weight loss after surgery tend to emerge around six months after the operation (Courcoulas et al. 2013). This seems to be a critical point at which the future direction of weight loss is set.

> You are always going to have that dramatic weight loss for a few months and that gives you the break to allow you to address your relationship with food. It's so important to use that time well to make new habits and change your mindset.
>
> TG, 16 months post bypass

If you imagine your weight loss journey as a climbing frame, the surgery itself gives you a leg up so you can get a foothold, but to keep moving or avoid falling, it's the next step that counts.

What causes weight regain or poor weight loss?

There isn't a straightforward or simple answer to this. It's the same mix of factors that are responsible for causing obesity in the first place – there isn't one single answer; it's a combination of factors that interact with each other. The different factors split into:

1) physical/surgical: hormone changes, surgical factors, e.g. size of pouch
2) psychological: changes in mental health, life events and challenges
3) behavioural: certain eating patterns (e.g. loss-of-control eating and grazing), non-adherence to the bariatric eating plan.

Although there is usually a combination of factors which cause weight regain or poor weight loss, people tend to fall into two extremes in terms of how they react to it. They blame themselves or they blame the surgery. Both these approaches tend to lead to inaction and prevent people from re-engaging with behaviour change. If people blame the surgery for weight regain (i.e. "There's something wrong with the operation") then they can just focus on finding another surgical "answer" to fix it, but it isn't that easy to find. Alternatively, if people blame themselves ("It's my fault, I'm a complete failure"), this can be very distressing and can trigger emotional eating patterns or old dieting behaviours of denial, restriction and deprivation, which are unsustainable.

Differences between weight maintainers and regainers

Some researchers found that when the six-month "honeymoon period" following bariatric surgery was over, people generally split into one of three groups, which the study defined as:

1) weight maintainers
2) weight regainers who were actively engaged in trying to lose weight
3) those who regained some weight but were not actively engaged in weight loss.

The authors of the study (Lynch 2016) identified some key differences between the three groups, as shown in Figure 12.1.

Another study, which followed people for over five years after having gastric bypass surgery, compared people who regained weight with

	Maintainers	Regained but losing weight	Regained
Hunger and fullness	Low levels of hunger; do not eat beyond fullness	Increased frequency of wanting to eat when not hungry; pay attention to fullness cues	Hunger between meals; fullness is short-lived; eat beyond fullness
Relationship with food	New relationship; food is not my "friend"; food "doesn't control me"	Aware of new vs old relationship with food; struggle to maintain new relationship	Retain pre-surgery relationship with food; food is "friend", "comfort" and used for coping
Habit formation	New habits formed and consistently used	Some "old habits" return and must be managed; most new habits maintained	Few new strategies for weight loss maintenance developed or implemented
Awareness of eating	Highly aware of behaviour and weight	Awareness of eating behaviour and increased awareness of behaviours that lead to weight gain	Less aware of portion sizes; weight or eating changes

Figure 12.1 Behavioural differences between the groups

Adapted from Lynch (2016).

Which group do you fall into?

Which behaviours do you recognise?

those that maintained weight. Those that regained weight tended to have a poor quality diet with excessive calories, snacks and sweets. They also had a sedentary lifestyle and tended to have missed follow-up appointments (Freire et al. 2012). Positive eating and activity habits provide you with a safety net that reduces the risk of weight regain.

Psychological responses to weight regain

The emotional reactions to weight regain obviously vary but often involve feelings of anxiety and self-criticism. These feelings of anxiety tend to happen because people feel out of control of their weight as it starts to creep up again. These feelings of anxiety can be overwhelming and make it difficult for people to engage in making small changes to get back on track. When people feel anxious, they tend to make predictions about worse case scenarios, for example, "I've completely blown it, my weight is just going to continue going up now and I'm going to end up back at square one". Remember, these are thoughts driven by anxiety, not facts. Usually people are terrible at making accurate predictions, too! These anxious thoughts get in the way of focusing and taking control by making small changes.

People can sometimes become very self-critical about any weight regain or poor weight loss after surgery. The problem with being your own worst critic is that it tends to make people feel terrible about themselves. This often leads to low mood, which in turn is associated with low motivation and activity. The thing that is supposed to motivate you actually has the opposite effect. Rather than being self-critical, try to step back and think about how you would speak to someone else in a similar situation. Try to find a compassionate, encouraging voice and acknowledge your effort so far and the fact that you are trying to do something that is difficult and challenging. Continuing to verbally punish yourself is a distraction and will not help you to start focusing on what you can do now to change your situation.

Some people also describe feeling ashamed that others may have noticed their weight regain. This can be particularly difficult if someone received lots of compliments and attention when they were initially losing weight. It is possible that you are more conscious of your weight regain than other people are. It may also be an opportunity to seek support and ask them to help you get back on track.

Although you may not have lost as much weight as you were hoping to after surgery, you may have stabilised your weight rather than continuing to put weight on. Your weight is still likely to be lower than it would have been without surgery. It's important to recognise that maintaining a stable weight is an achievement in its own right, especially for those people whose weight was continuously increasing previously.

Importance of seeking help from your bariatric service

When people have struggled to lose weight after surgery or have regained weight, they can sometimes avoid going to the bariatric clinic because of a sense of shame or worry that they will be "told off". Some people worry that they will appear ungrateful for "wasting an opportunity" that they have been given or that they are "letting the team down", and this can lead to avoidance, too. It is important to remember that the staff working in the bariatric service are there to help you and will be used to people struggling with their weight after bariatric surgery. As discussed before, weight regain happens to 20–30% of people. We know that weight management is complex and challenging – if life after bariatric surgery was plain sailing, there would be no need for services to provide follow-up! Furthermore, professionals generally choose to work in bariatric surgery because they are sensitive to the issues experienced by people with weight problems.

Is it possible to lose weight again? What is realistic?

Yes! It is only in the last few years that there has been research looking at whether it is possible or realistic to reverse the trend and lose regained weight after bariatric surgery. This means that there is limited data, but the information available does suggest that it is possible. This has been my clinical experience, too.

One study (Himes et al. 2015) found that people who had regained more than 15% of their weight were able to lose weight during a six-week group. They found that there were strong patterns of emotional eating amongst people who experienced weight regain or poor weight loss after surgery. They found that binge eating, emotional eating and grazing reduced after the group, and that the reduction in these behaviours was associated with weight loss. This information is useful because it highlights the type of behaviours that need to be targeted because they are associated with weight regain.

Although it's obviously important to re-engage with making changes to your eating patterns and behaviour in order to lose weight, it's equally important to focus on making these changes to improve your psychological wellbeing. Distress about eating patterns is related to poor psychological health and wellbeing, so making changes can lead to positive improvements in this area, too. It can help people to regain a sense of control and achievement.

It feels desperate when I feel that I have lost control of my eating. But, whereas before it felt desperate *and* hopeless now it's desperate but I know that I can regain control. It no longer feels like the end of the world and there's a stopping point. Before surgery it was like, 'This is where I am, there's nothing you can do . . . you are what you are, so keep eating'. Now I think, 'Accept where you are and just wait for the moment you need where you can get the foothold to start again'. Maybe you can't do anything in that moment but it doesn't mean you can't do something in the next moment. I know for a fact that if I eat the way I'm meant to eat and stick to the guidelines then I will get to the weight that I'm meant to be. Before surgery I used to believe it was hopeless and that whatever I did it was never going to work. Now I 100% know if I do what I am supposed to do then I will be a reasonable weight.

SG, 4 years post bypass

Even though I've gained some weight again after surgery, I've noticed that it hasn't been as drastic. It feels like the extra weight gain is something that you can lose. For example, if I gained 20kg before surgery then I would think, 'Oh god, it's going to take ages to lose it' and it would feel completely unmanageable. Whereas after surgery if you've gained 4–5kg then you know that there's something that you can do to lose the weight. I would just give up before because it would feel impossible.

AD, 4 years post bypass

In the next section, we start to focus on the things that you can do to start addressing your current weight issues. The first step involves making sense of what has led to either suboptimal weight loss or weight regain. Without this understanding, it is difficult for people to make changes that are likely to be effective. You have to identify the problem to work out the solution.

Identifying the reasons for weight regain – doing your own assessment

Mapping out your weight loss trajectory to gather information

If you map out your weight loss trajectory over time, you can start to see where your weight loss started to plateau or where regain started. You can then start to investigate this to gather information about your different phases of weight loss. Focusing on the speed and direction of your weight loss over time by joining the dots up in a graph is very informative. The aim is to identify when, how and where the pattern of weight loss started to change. For some people, this can be a gradual, steady weight regain or for others, it can be a sudden weight gain. For example, a woman who had lost 43kg at 18 months post bypass regained 17kg over a six-month period. The reason for this weight regain was that she'd had to go back to the town where she was born for the funeral of her grandmother and then stayed there for a month. This was the first time that she had been back there since having surgery. She identified a number of factors that had contributed to her weight regain. She had stopped planning her meals and she had accepted foods that she wouldn't normally eat as she was too embarrassed to decline foods for risk of offending people. By being very clear about the trigger for the weight regain and the behaviours that had changed, it meant that she was able

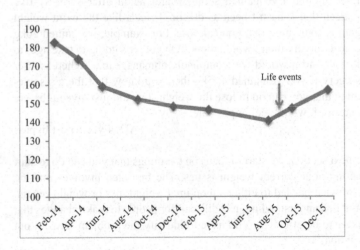

Figure 12.2 Using a weight loss trajectory graph to help identify triggers for weight regain

to identify the behaviours that are crucial in helping her stay on track (i.e. planning her meals and sticking to her plan regardless of other people offering tempting foods). She was able to see how quickly not sticking to these behaviours affected her weight. She was also able to think about the plans she needed to put in place for the next time she went back to her home town in order to avoid weight regain.

When you look at your weight trajectory, ask yourself the following questions:

- Was there a gradual increase in your weight or a certain point where it increased significantly?
- At what point did your weight change? What was happening in your life around this time?
- What happened to your eating and activity levels at this point? What did you start doing and what did you stop doing?
- What were you doing when you were happiest with your eating/ weight loss?

You could also try asking close friends or family what changes they have noticed over time, as it can sometimes be difficult to spot changes yourself, especially if there has been a gradual change.

Once you have worked out what some of the shifts and changes are that you need to make, you can use some of the resources from the earlier chapters to help you with these. The areas discussed in these earlier chapters, for example, regular eating, planning meals and managing emotional eating, apply to people who have had their operation as well as people who are pre surgery.

Self-monitoring your eating and activity

It is important to get information about your eating (and activity levels) so you can look at what patterns you may have slipped into. This will help you work out what the problems are. In addition, the process of monitoring often leads to people naturally making changes as their awareness increases.

You can use the resources in Chapter 2 to help you monitor and assess your eating.

Aiming for weight stabilisation as a first step

People often discount or forget that stabilising their weight is an important goal and is an achievement in its own right. The natural tendency is for weight to drift upwards. It's important to stabilise so that you can then either accept this is the weight you are going to work at maintaining, or think about what you need to do to move into a weight loss phase.

Getting ready to make changes

Before you can start to make changes, you may have to build your motivation again. Part of this involves believing that what you do will make a difference. It's important to set yourself small, achievable goals so that you get a sense that what you are doing is working and is manageable. Try to avoid panicking or trying anything too radical (e.g. the latest fad diet). We are aiming for slow and steady changes that you can maintain.

> In the first 18 months I was very engaged. Food was something to keep me going. I would eat just to give my body fuel. From the moment I wasn't at home and in control of my routine or environment anymore, things started to change. I lost control . . . the picking came back and suddenly I was eating the top of a pizza, picking at the inside of fish and chips . . . my choices started to change. There were changes over time . . . now the food went back to being my comfort, not a fuel. I've started to make small changes again and it has helped raise my awareness of the choices I'm making. I've started thinking about how I am serving food and putting some limits back in place again.
>
> AC, 26 months post bypass

Think about some of the changes you made either before or just after surgery. What worked for you then?

It can sometimes be difficult to get started with changes again as people automatically tend to think about things that they have to stop doing or do less of. This can trigger a feeling of resentment or deprivation. You may find it more helpful to focus on the things you could do more of rather than what you need to do less of at this stage, for example, focusing on eating more protein foods rather than decreasing carbohydrates.

Strategies

The next section includes an overview of various strategies that you can use to get back on track. It would be unwise and unrealistic to try to implement all of these at once! They are listed below so that you can pick one to start changing – it doesn't matter where you start or how small the change is. Give yourself credit for engaging with the process and regaining a sense of control over your eating and weight. Most of the strategies outlined are ones which have been previously discussed in this book so they may sound familiar – the skills for getting back on track are no different to those which you previously used to help you to start make changes. Summaries of the strategies are outlined, alongside information on which earlier chapter includes more detailed information.

Refreshing your knowledge

- Reminding yourself about the bariatric plan: have you got the right information?
- Do you know what are the most appropriate foods? Do you know what a "typical" bariatric eating plan looks like?
- Do you know what the golden rules are?
- Do you know what the appropriate portion size is?

Re-establishing an eating plan

- This involves eating regularly and working out a meal structure throughout the day.
- Work out a meal plan. You could plan one day at a time or it could be for the week ahead.
- Check your portion sizes and the plates you use.
- Check your food choices – in particular, are you having enough protein?
- Use the golden rules.
- Think about how you do your food shopping – does this work for you or do you need to reconsider how you shop?

Strategies to address these issues are in Chapter 2.

Identifying any problem eating

Particular patterns to look out for include:

- grazing
- emotional eating
- loss-of-control eating.

Strategies to address these specific patterns are included in Chapter 3 and Chapter 7.

Communicating changes to others

Do the people you live with help you stay on track, or do they play a role in sending you off track?

As you start to introduce changes to your eating and routine, it is important to discuss and inform these with people you are close to. Just the process of letting others know about the plan is a good starting point – it makes your intentions clear and makes you more accountable. The ideal scenario is that people will help you and support you to make these changes. However, you may also need to be prepared to make the changes alone; obviously, this requires focus and determination.

Physical activity

Some options for increasing your physical activity include:

- walking regularly (you could consider joining a walking group)
- changing an aspect of in your routine, e.g. walking rather than catching the bus
- reducing your sedentary behaviour – try to remember to stand up regularly
- considering re-engaging with any previous activities
- signing up for an activity or exercise class
- thinking about what time of day is best for you to engage in physical activity.

Other options are included in Chapter 9.

Dealing with any underlying issues/stressors

When you step back and analyse what difficulties may have contributed to your weight regain, sometimes the weight regain is a consequence of another problem.

Other examples of issues include:

- bereavement
- caring for others
- stress at work
- breakdown of relationships
- worry about finances
- relocation, changing job or moving home
- illness (self or family member).

These are examples of situations that are likely to send your eating off track or shift your focus. It is important to backtrack to problem-solve the trigger situation. This means that you are addressing the cause (life events) as well as the consequences (eating). You may need to seek help from friends, family or healthcare professionals to work out some ways of addressing the underlying problem.

Support

Other sources of support include your bariatric team and joining a bariatric support group.

Revisional surgery – other options

When people have unmet weight loss expectations after surgery or have regained weight, they may start to consider additional or revisional bariatric surgery. If you consider that obesity is a chronic condition then it is likely that people will need further treatment. Further surgery is something to consider very carefully. For some people their primary bariatric operation may not have been the best choice for them (e.g. having a gastric band is a very different experience to having a bypass) or may have happened at a difficult or challenging time in their life. Revisional surgery can be a reset opportunity and a fresh start. However, it is only worth considering further surgery if you know that you have the right tools and strategies in place, and that you have addressed any issues that have got in the way of your weight loss previously. You also need to consider whether this is the ideal point in your life to consider further surgery.

There is some evidence that people can lose additional weight with another bariatric operation. The most common options are conversion from gastric band to a sleeve gastrectomy/gastric bypass or from sleeve gastrectomy to a bypass. It is challenging to calculate the amount of weight that someone is likely to lose with their second procedure, but it is likely to be less than they lost with their primary bariatric operation. It is also important to bear in mind that the risks of surgery are higher with revisional surgery.

Summary

Unmet weight loss expectations and weight regain can be very upsetting and difficult to cope with. However, it's important not to abandon hope and to become paralysed by self-blame or self-criticism – if you reassess your behaviour and start making some changes then it is possible to manage your weight and to feel better about yourself.

References

Aftab, H., et al., 2014. Five-year outcome after gastric bypass for morbid obesity in a Norwegian cohort. *Surgery for Obesity and Related Diseases*, 10 (1), 71–78.

Courcoulas, A.P., et al., 2013. Weight change and health outcomes at 3 years after bariatric surgery among individuals with severe obesity. *Journal of the American Medical Association*, 1521 3(22), 1–10.

De Hollanda, A., et al., 2014. Patterns of weight loss response following gastric bypass and sleeve gastrectomy. *Obesity Surgery*, 25, 1177–1183.

Freire, R.H., et al., 2012. Food quality, physical activity, and nutritional follow-up as determinant of weight regain after Roux-en-Y gastric bypass. *Nutrition*, 28 (1), 53–58.

Himes, S.M., et al., 2015. Stop regain: a pilot psychological intervention for bariatric patients experiencing weight regain. *Obesity Surgery*, 25 (5), 922–927.

Lynch, A., 2016. "When the honeymoon is over, the real work begins": Gastric bypass patients' weight loss trajectories and dietary change experiences. *Social Science and Medicine*, 151, 241–249.

Sheets, C.S., et al., 2014. Post-operative psychosocial predictors of outcome in bariatric surgery. *Obesity Surgery*, 25 (2), 330–345.

Index

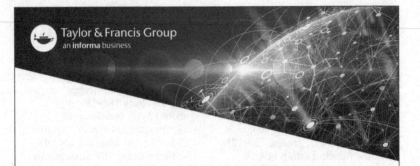